Feeding
Toddlers

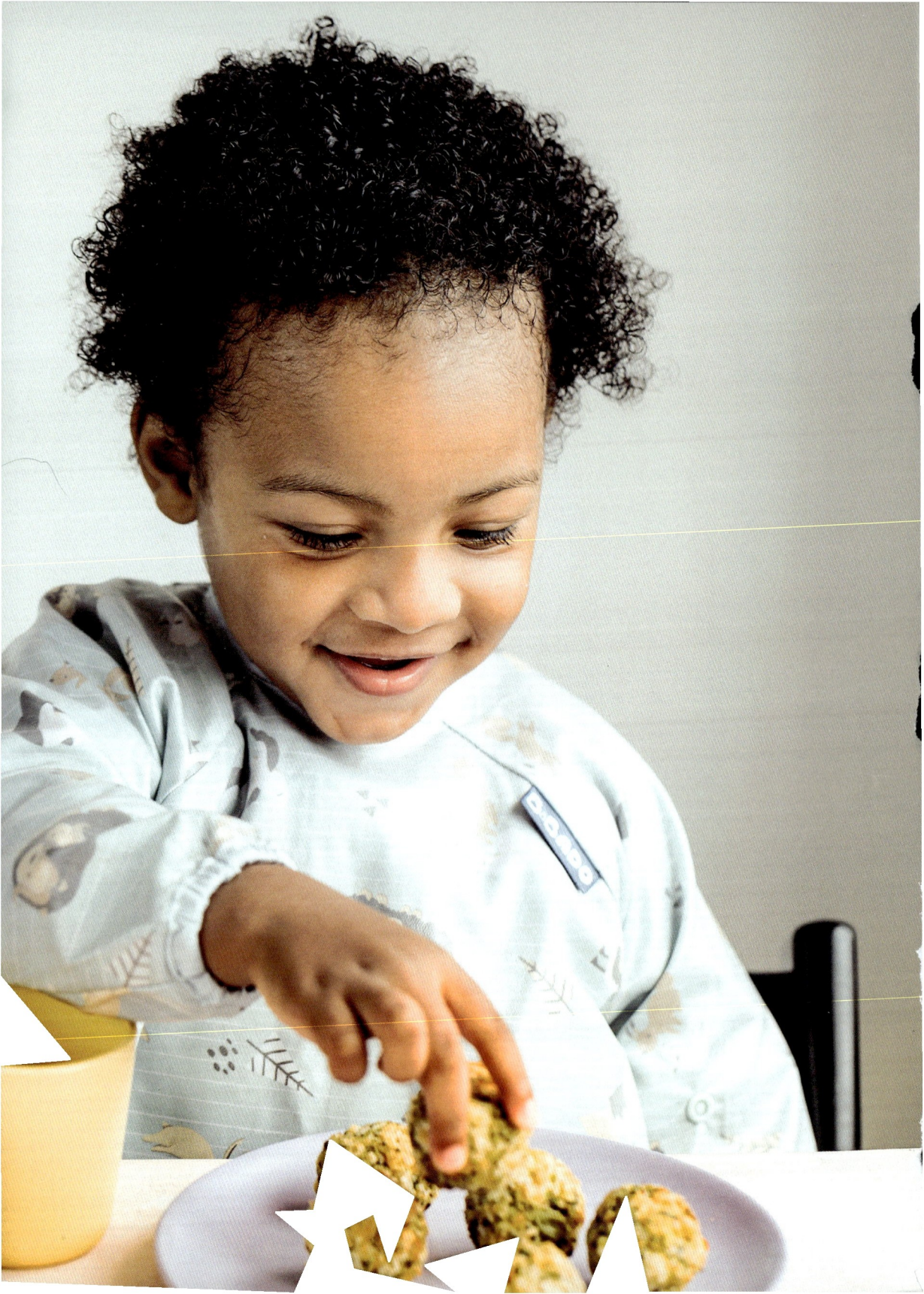

Feeding Toddlers

The Complete Guide to Maintaining Nutrition *and* Variety *with* Easy Family Meals

Simone Ward

Creator of **ZAYNE'S PLATE**

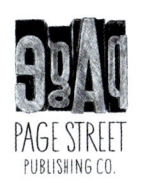

PAGE STREET
PUBLISHING CO.

PAGE STREET
PUBLISHING CO.

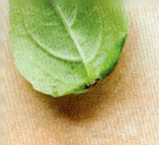

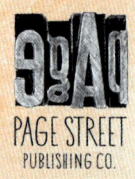

Copyright © 2024 Simone Ward

First published in 2024 by
Page Street Publishing Co.
27 Congress Street, Suite 1511
Salem, MA 01970
www.pagestreetpublishing.com

All rights reserved. No part of this book may be reproduced or used, in any form or by any means, electronic or mechanical, without prior permission in writing from the publisher.

Distributed by Macmillan, sales in Canada by The Canadian Manda Group.

28 27 26 25 24   1 2 3 4 5

ISBN-13: 979-8-89003-005-4

Library of Congress Control Number: 2023948959

Cover and book design by Rosie Stewart for Page Street Publishing Co.
Photography by Kimberly Espinel
Food styling by Alicja Sieronski
Prop styling by Kimberly Espinel, Alicja Sieronski and Simone Ward

Printed and bound in the United States of America

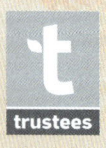

t trustees
Page Street Publishing protects our planet by donating to nonprofits like The Trustees, which focuses on local land conservation.

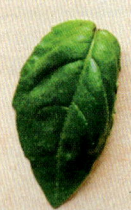

Dedication

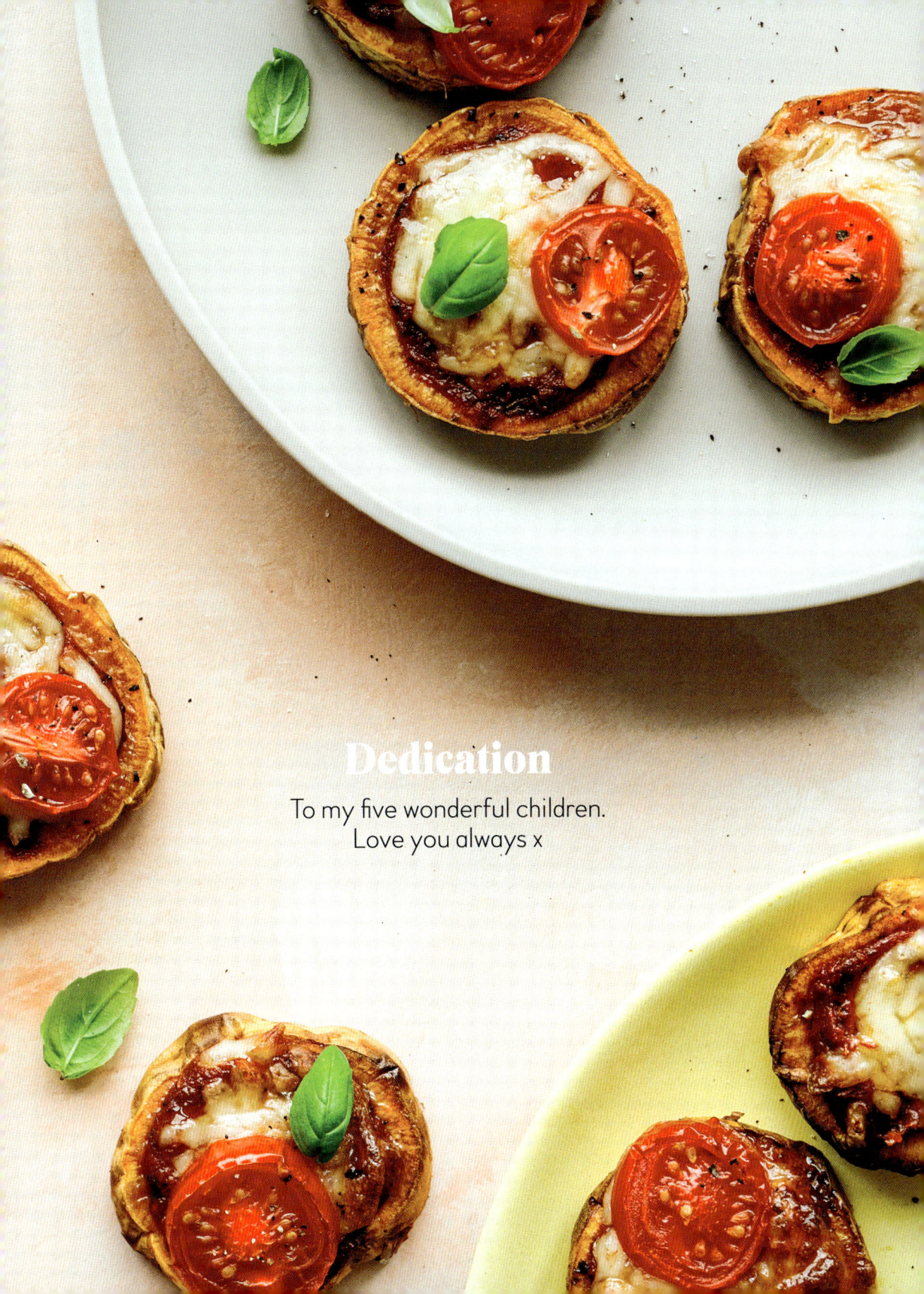

To my five wonderful children.
Love you always x

Introduction 9

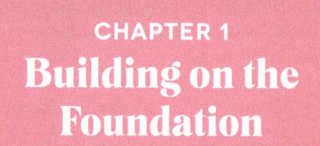

CHAPTER 1
Building on the Foundation

What to Expect When Feeding Kids 1–4 Years Old 11
Picky Eating & Sane Solutions 11
Choking Hazard Guidelines (Ages 1–4) 16
How to Introduce & Manage Sugar in a Realistic Way 18
Age Suitability & Portion Size 21
Common Questions 21

CHAPTER 2
Smart Snacking

Introducing Snacks 27
Healthy Snacks for Toddlers & Kids 27
Simple Snack Building Formula 28
Scheduling Snacks 28
Tips for Stress-Free Snack Times 29
Easy Balanced Snack Examples 30
Speedy Snack Cheat Sheet 31

CHAPTER 3
Making the Most of Breakfast

Whole-Wheat Protein Blender Waffles 37
Toddler-Friendly Nut-Free Granola 38
Broccoli & Cheese Sheet Pan Eggs 41
Fluffy Applesauce Pancakes 42
Blueberry & Banana French Toast Bake 45
Easy Peachy Smoothie Bowl 46
Sweet Potato Breakfast Hash 49
Breakfast Banana Cake Cups 50
Savory Cheddar Waffles 53
Iron-Rich Banana & Cashew Oatmeal 54

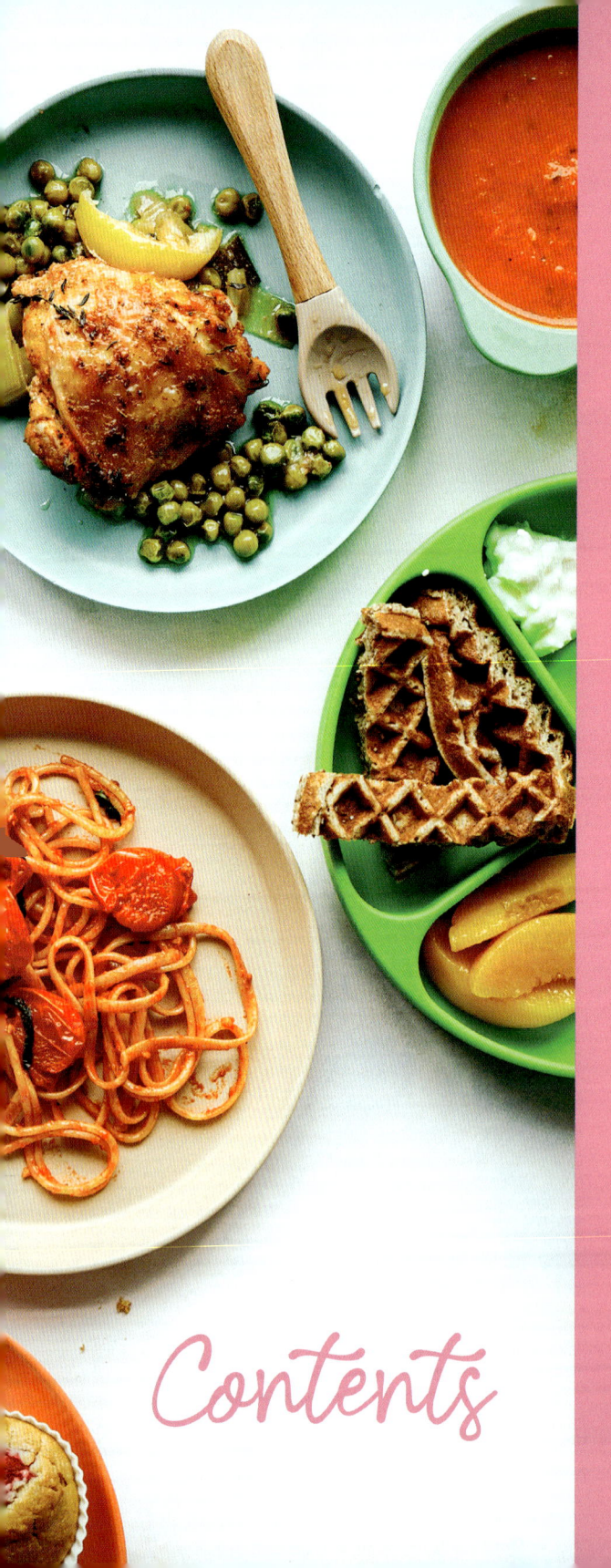

Contents

CHAPTER 4
Nutritious & Delicious Mains that Little Ones Will Love

20-Minute Iron-Rich Tomato Soup 59
Smoky Honey Chicken Drumsticks 60
Oven-Baked Turkey & Spinach Meatballs 63
Sweet Potato Mini Pizzas 66
Crispy Salmon Bites 69
Hearty Mexican Chicken Quesadillas 71
Stovetop Pumpkin Mac & Cheese 75
Lamb Kofta & Tzatziki Dip 76
Lazy Lasagna Soup 79
Curried Lentil & Veggie Soup 82
Speedy Cherry Tomato Spaghetti 85
Shrimp Cakes 86
Falafel Patties 89
10-Minute Peanut Noodles 90
Quick-Cook Sausage & Pepper Stew 93
Avocado Egg Salad 94
Lemony Chicken & Leek Sheet Pan 97
Crispy Sweet Corn Fritters 98
Spinach & Cod Mild Coconut Curry 101
Chunky Veggie Pasta Bake 102

CHAPTER 5
Something Different on the Side

Crispy Zucchini Fries 107
Cheesy Garlic Bread 108
Sautéed Green Beans 111
Easy Garlic Noodles 112
Parmesan Crusted Roasties 115
Lemon Garlic Dip 116

Eggy Bread Rolls 119
Broccoli Mashed Potatoes 120
Crispy Smoky Roasted Eggplant 123
Cinnamon Roasted Sweet Potatoes 124
Homemade Marinara Dipping Sauce 127

CHAPTER 6
Make-Ahead Snacks & Bakes

Orange & Raspberry Muffins 131
No-Bake Multigrain Cereal Bars 132
Bite-Size Fruity Cheesecake Strudels 135
Iron-Rich Almond & Coconut Cookies 138
Pumpkin Pie Mini Muffins 141
Cheesy Broccoli Balls 142
Apple & Carrot Snack Bars 145
Lemon & Blueberry Yogurt Muffins 146
Chocolate Oat Bites 149

CHAPTER 7
Meal Plans

How the Meal Plan Works 152
Meal Plan Week 1 154
Meal Plan Week 2 156
Meal Plan Week 3 158
Meal Plan Week 4 160

American/British Ingredient Translations 162
Acknowledgments 162
About the Author 163
Index 164

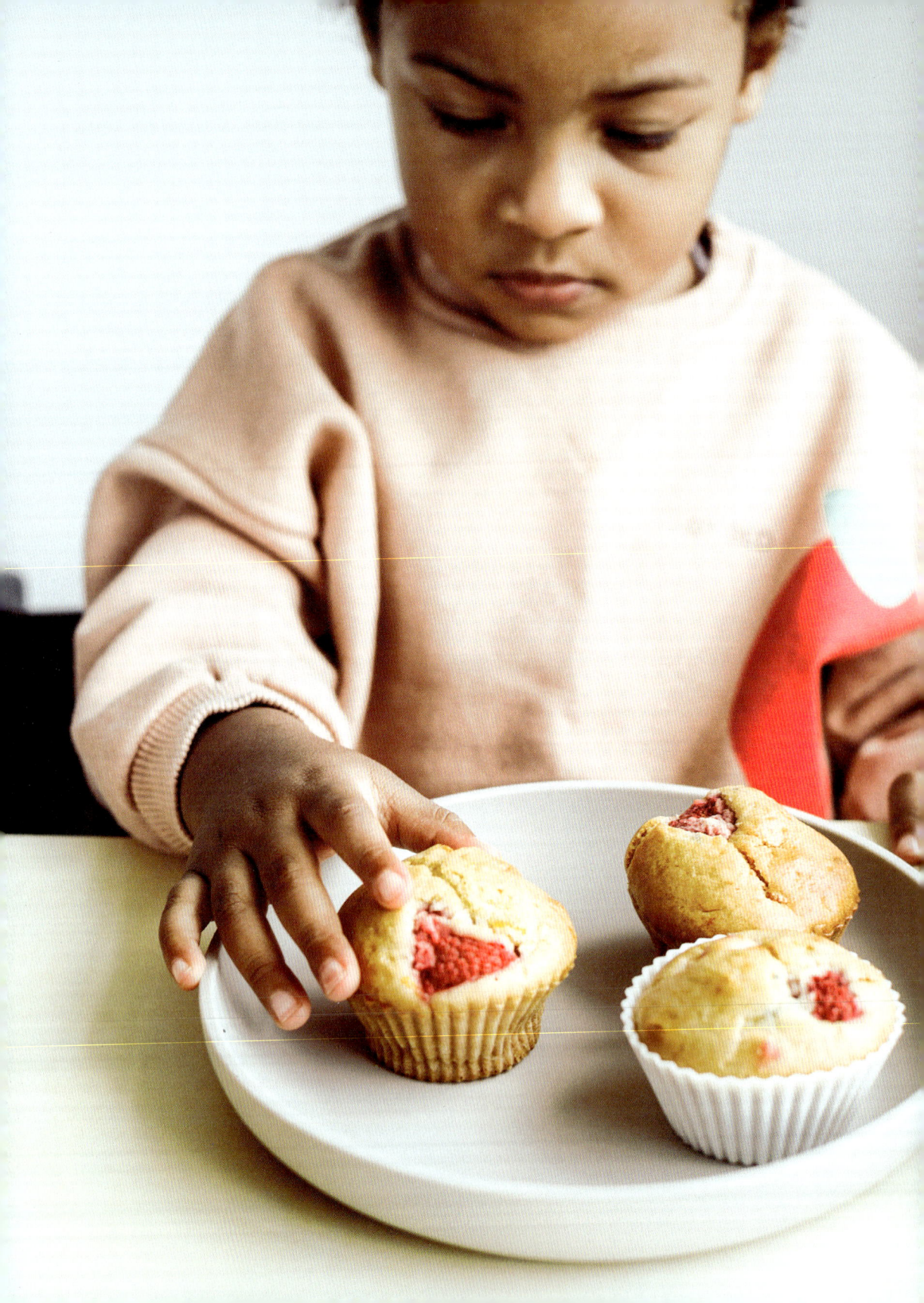

Introduction

Welcome—I'm so glad you are here! I'm Simone, a mom of five, food writer and founder of the popular Instagram blog @zaynesplate, where I create and share content about the food I feed my children. I specialize in creating nutritious recipes and meal ideas for babies, toddlers and kids. This my second cookbook, which focuses primarily on feeding toddlers, and I am so excited to share some more of my tried-and-true, family-friendly recipes with you, as well as information on how you can navigate those tricky toddler feeding years.

My main goal is to provide you with ideas and strategies that are realistic and easily applied to everyday life—the last thing I want is to overwhelm you with too much information or give you recipes that are complicated and leave you feeling chained to the stove. I am all about the simple meals that appeal to both toddlers and adults and focus on flavor and nutrition, but in an unintimidating way that won't overwhelm your kids.

The bulk of this book is my recipes. One thing I am known for is providing nutritious yet uncomplicated meals, which are easy to prepare using simplified cooking methods. Here you will find a wide variety of recipes and flavor combinations that will help you keep mealtimes interesting and avoid falling into a rut. Your family will love these meals, and you will not need to cook separately for your toddler—one meal for the whole family is always the goal!

I have also included four weekly meal plans (each one including meals for seven days) to help you incorporate the recipes from this book into your day-to-day life. This book will not collect dust, and the meal plans will help you to stay consistent in preparing flavorful home-cooked meals for your family. Of course, you may still wish to rotate meals and family favorites around to suit your loved ones, so be realistic and understanding with your goals as you give them a try.

Besides the fantastic recipes and meal plans, you will also find practical information that will support you in some key areas in feeding your toddler. Whether it's figuring out how to introduce snacks or how to manage sugar intake, I have sifted through all the unnecessary information and advice and provided you with the most important evidence-based strategies and recommendations that will enable you to support your toddler in making the most of their appetite and creating a realistic and healthy relationship with sugar and food in general.

And let's not forget picky eating! I am passionate about taking a gentle approach to feeding toddlers, especially when it comes to tackling picky eating. We will all likely go through this tricky phase, and although this book isn't an extensive picky eating guide, I have touched on the most common issues to help you support your toddler in a stress-free way.

Lastly, I want to reassure you that you are not alone on this challenging journey of feeding your toddler, and almost all of us have been or are currently going through the same issues and phases. I hope that this book will be an invaluable resource for you and encourage you to relax and develop confidence in both yourself and your toddler at mealtimes. This journey doesn't have to be stressful because believe it or not, feeding toddlers can be simple and enjoyable! I hope this book helps you and your family!

Simone Ward

CHAPTER 1

Building on the Foundation

In my first book, *Baby-Led Weaning Made Easy*, I primarily focused on feeding babies and the introduction of solids. That book's approach prioritized the ways that we can lay down the foundations for adventurous eating and help babies get a kick-start on having a good relationship with food. My approach to feeding toddlers naturally follows this, and my main goal is to continue to build on this foundation and give toddlers and young kids the tools they need to navigate eating in their big, new world that they are so very keen to explore!

Feeding toddlers can be vastly different to feeding babies—just as we feel we have got the hang of things, our babies suddenly move into a new stage of development and become independent(ish) toddlers. What often comes as a surprise is that things can change, sometimes dramatically, and feeding toddlers can often prove to be very tricky! Now, in my opinion, toddlers are great. It's a wonderful age for exploration and development, and it's a beautiful thing to watch them navigate their newfound independence. But I'd be lying if I said that feeding toddlers was effortlessly easy. There are good days and weeks, but there can also be some challenging times—it's very much like a roller coaster for both us and them!

In this chapter, I walk you through some of the things you can expect when feeding toddlers, and why what might seem like an issue isn't an issue at all. Even when issues do arise, there is a lot we can do to support our kids in moving through them. It's hard to know what lies ahead, but I hope this chapter will help to prepare you for the more common changes and challenges.

What to Expect When Feeding Kids 1-4 Years Old

During their first year, babies experience the fastest period of growth that their bodies will ever go through—they typically triple their birth weight! Due to this rapid growth, babies use up a ton of energy, so it's not unusual for them to have ferocious appetites—whether it be for breastmilk, formula or solids. Once baby turns one, growth starts to slow down significantly, and your now toddler, who may have previously eaten everything you placed in front of them, starts eating less. Please don't panic if this happens; you are not doing anything wrong. This appetite adjustment is completely normal and to be expected.

Of course, this doesn't happen to all toddlers, and if your toddler's appetite has remained the same, that is perfectly fine too. It doesn't mean they are overeating or will gain more weight than they need to. It's also normal for their appetites to fluctuate, and they might eat a ton of food one day and eat like a bird the next, or maybe they pack in a lot of food at breakfast and then it tapers off throughout the day—again, totally normal. Ultimately, a kid's needs are ever changing, and there is so much that can impact their appetite, so if you do have a toddler who has developed a lower or unpredictable appetite, it doesn't necessarily mean that they have become a picky eater!

Picky Eating & Sane Solutions

Picky eating is something that can dominate our day-to-day lives and cause us a lot of worry. Not all toddlers become picky. Some will happily continue to eat a wide variety of foods, while many others will display at least some level of picky eating as they move through toddlerhood, and it can last longer for some kids than others.

What's important to understand is that picky eating is generally a normal developmental stage. You can do everything "right" and still have a toddler who becomes picky, so please don't blame yourself! What's most important is how we respond to picky eating and how we support toddlers in moving through what is typically a very normal and age-appropriate stage of development.

IS MY TODDLER PICKY?

There are a lot of misunderstandings around picky eating, and it can often leave us feeling confused and unsure about how to move forward. I first want to highlight some behaviors that are not typically signs of picky eating or something you need to worry about.

Your toddler is not picky just because they:

- eat less than they did as a baby.
- don't clear their plate or eat as much as you feel they should.
- frontload their calories and eat a lot at breakfast, but less as the day goes on.
- have an appetite that fluctuates day to day or meal to meal.
- have general preferences for certain foods or food groups.
- have some foods that they do not like.
- are slow to warm up to new foods.

As with anything, these things are not black and white, and it is possible that in some cases, the behaviors displayed above can be attributed to picky eating. But for the most part, they are not indicative of picky eating or poor eating habits in general.

With normal picky eating, toddlers may display more actively resistive behaviors toward food. I have listed some of these more common signs below, but every toddler is different and will often display their own quirky signs of pickiness that are specific to their circumstances.

Signs of normal toddler picky eating:

- Refusing a wide variety of foods
- Rejecting foods they once loved
- Rejecting foods if they aren't prepared in a certain way (e.g., you cut their sandwich wrong)
- Refusing to try new foods
- Showing little enjoyment in food
- Willing to skip meals if preferred foods are unavailable
- Eating a different meal from the rest of the family
- Eating a limited amount of food
- Liking something one day but not the next

I want to reiterate that this kind of picky eating is normal! Learning to eat is a process, and it comes with many ups and downs. As frustrating as it feels while we're going through it, most kids do grow out of it and begin to accept a wider range of foods in time.

REASONS BEHIND TODDLER PICKY EATING

There are many things that may contribute to picky eating. Below, I have touched on a wide range of these reasons, along with some ways to help your toddler work through them. Not all will apply at the same time (if at all), so don't feel like you must implement all the strategies at once—tackle any issues one step at a time and at a pace that doesn't overwhelm you or your toddler.

Normal Toddler Development

One reason picky eating can emerge is down to typical toddler development that occurs between the ages of 1 and 4. During this time, toddlers learn to walk and talk and suddenly they are busy bees—always on the move and enthusiastically exploring everything their world has to offer. By exploring this independence, they quickly realize that they are their own person who can say no to something, and with that comes the need for more control. Choosing what to eat (or what not to eat) is a normal and expected part of their development, and mealtimes are the easiest and most convenient place for them to assert their independence and maintain some control in their day-to-day lives.

No Division of Responsibility

Whenever I talk about navigating picky eating, I always start with the Division of Responsibility (DoR). Developed by Ellen Satter, the DoR is an evidence-based feeding method that allows parents to set appropriate boundaries around food and mealtimes that work alongside children (of any age) to give them the space they need to learn and trust in their own hunger and fullness cues by providing an inviting and no-pressure environment that allows them to explore both new and familiar foods.

Toddlers are naturally skilled at knowing what their bodies need and when, and research has shown that to effectively tackle picky eating, we must first allow them to nurture this skill by giving them the opportunity to eat intuitively and have complete control over their food intake. This doesn't mean they get to dictate which foods you serve them, but they must have the complete freedom to choose what and how much to eat from the meals and snacks that you provide.

The DoR works in practice by assigning specific roles to the parent and the child and advises that both parties act only with these boundaries.

Those roles are as follows:

- The parent is responsible for what foods to offer and when and where to offer them.
- The child is responsible for whether or not to eat and how much to eat of the foods offered.

The best way to put DoR into practice is to have set meal and snack times so that your toddler will always know that there will be food coming and put zero pressure on them to eat. As I explore the day-to-day causes of picky eating and how we can work through them, I do so with the DoR in mind, ensuring that all these methods will support your child in harnessing their internal food regulation and help you to cultivate positive attitudes about eating and food. Let's create a mealtime environment that is free from pressure and prevent food battles around picky eating and the stress that often follows!

Grazing and Lack of Mealtime Routine

Mealtime schedules are arguably one of the most important pieces of the puzzle when it comes to feeding kids. Toddlers have small tummies that can only hold so much food, and as such, they need regular opportunities to eat. With that said, having unstructured and unlimited access to food typically results in them grazing all day and filling up on snacks between meals. As a result, they come to the table with a low appetite and little enthusiasm for the nourishing meals you have prepared. Creating an eating schedule that offers meals and snacks at regular intervals (usually every 2 to 3 hours), means that both you and your toddler can relax in the knowledge that there will be several opportunities to eat throughout the day, and if they are not hungry for the meal or snack you have provided, another will be along soon.

Example Toddler Feeding Schedule:

MORNING	AFTERNOON	EVENING
7:00 Breakfast	12:00 Lunch	6:00 Dinner
9:00 Snack	3:00 Snack	Bedtime Snack (optional)

Eating schedules will vary depending on your toddler's age and individual needs and may require some trial and error when it comes to naps and leaving the house. The table to the left is just one example, but feel free to adjust it to suit your toddler's routine or your family's lifestyle.

Overwhelming Portion Sizes

Plating up large portions of food can be overwhelming and off-putting for some toddlers, which can result in disengagement at the table, food throwing and food refusal. If you think this could be the case for your toddler, try starting them off with much smaller portions and top them up as needed.

Milk Intake

Drinking a lot of milk can have a direct impact on your toddler's appetite and displace other foods in their diet. Additionally, excess intake of animal and/or plant-based milks has been linked to an increased risk of iron deficiency, and as such, should be limited to 16 ounces (480 ml) per day. If you are breastfeeding, you can continue offering breastmilk on demand, so long as it doesn't interfere with your toddler's appetite for solid foods.

Pressure and Bribery

It's easy to get caught up in using pressure and bribery techniques to get toddlers to eat—we've all been there! But when kids feel under pressure, they can become more inclined to eat less or reject foods altogether, and mealtimes can feel like a battleground.

Pressure comes in many forms, more classically by implementing rules such as taking a "no thank you bite" or withholding dessert until all the food on their plate has been eaten. But it can also come in the form of positive reinforcement, such as actively encouraging them to eat during mealtimes by cheering them on or whooping when they try new foods—although it comes from a loving place, it can often have the opposite effect over time and can teach kids to override their own hunger and satiety cues in order to receive praise or please others.

Sometimes pressure strategies can appear to be working in the short term, but what tends to happen is that it backfires and causes more issues long term and only serves to increase picky eating and food refusal over time. We can help our toddlers to enjoy mealtimes and eat more by creating a positive eating environment that is free from pressure, allowing them to eat and explore foods instinctively and respecting their choice to stop eating when they feel full.

Teething

Without a doubt, teething is one the biggest reasons for a toddler's appetite plummeting. All types of teething can affect a baby or toddler's appetite, but toddlers in particular will begin to cut their molars, which are the teeth we use to chew and grind down food. As such, they can find eating especially painful.

Reluctance to eat during this time is completely normal, and your toddler's appetite will likely return once the tooth they are cutting has erupted and the inflammation on their gums has calmed down. In the meantime, you can help them by offering soft and easy to chew foods, such as oatmeal, scrambled eggs and soft bread, or cold foods, such as homemade popsicles and smoothies. Some toddlers will also enjoy gnawing on hard, resistive foods, such as a mango pit or corn on the cob.

Tiredness

Overtired toddlers will not fare well at the table. This can happen at any time of the day, but dinner is often the usual time and place for tired meltdowns. If this happens often in your home, you might find it helpful to offer dinner earlier—even 30 minutes can make a big difference to a tired toddler!

Not Eating with Family

Many toddlers are less likely to eat if they are alone. Eating together can help them to eat more and explore new foods. Children learn and are encouraged by watching those around them, so sitting with them and being a role model eater is invaluable. Eating together also helps to take the focus off the food, and instead puts precedence on reconnecting and enjoying each other's company, which puts less pressure on both you and your toddler for them to eat.

Lack of Variety

The variety of foods your toddler is willing to eat naturally reduces with picky eating, and sometimes, in the quest to ensure that they are happy and fed we fall into a cycle of repeating the same meals and snacks over and over, just to ensure that their tummies are full. While this is completely understandable, before we know it, they are being exposed to less and less variety as time goes by. The thing is, toddlers are unlikely to broaden their palates and try new foods if they are not exposed to them. Learning to like new or challenging foods takes time and the only way to help our kids along the way is to serve these foods regularly and on rotation with the foods we know they enjoy and will reliably eat. This doesn't mean we have to drastically cut down on offering our toddler's favorites, but ideally we want to resist the urge to repeat the same foods two days in a row (besides milk and leftovers) and aim to include more variety in our overall meal and snack rotation.

No Safe Foods

When offering your toddler new or challenging foods, are you offering a safe food too? Safe foods are foods that a picky toddler likes and will reliably eat, and by offering at least one safe food with every meal and snack we are ensuring that first, they will at least have something they can eat and enjoy so they won't leave the table hungry, and secondly, we are being considerate of their preferences, but not catering to them. This takes a lot of pressure off everyone by taking the focus off of what they may or may not eat during a meal and enabling them to explore foods instinctively and in their own time.

Let Them Make a Mess!

Micromanaging our toddlers' meals and interfering with the ways in which they choose to eat can prevent them from exploring in ways that lead to adventurous eating. First, toddlers can be messy—they love to play! Not only does this encourage them to try new foods and tolerate different textures, but it also helps them to learn the skills they need to eat, such as using utensils. If you struggle with mess, this can be a really challenging part of feeding, but instead of trying to prevent the mess altogether, try to instead focus on making the clean-up easier. Double up on bibs by layering a silicone catcher bib over a full coverage smock bib, lay a splash mat on the floor, and keep a jug of water nearby so you can easily rinse off those mucky hands before your toddler even leaves the table!

WHEN IT'S MORE THAN A PHASE

Sometimes, picky eating is more than just a phase, and things can fail to improve even when we implement all the recommended techniques. It could be that the range of foods your toddler will eat keeps narrowing and they are beginning to cut out entire food groups, or maybe they are refusing all solids, and will only drink milk no matter what you have tried. Maybe you have reached a point where your toddler's ability to socialize is being affected and visiting loved ones outside the home or going to parties has become stressful because of their picky eating. Sometimes kids need some additional support from outside sources, and this doesn't mean that either of you have failed. If you are in any way worried about your child's health, growth or development, do not hesitate to reach out to their doctor or a feeding specialist and access support.

FINAL THOUGHTS ON PICKY EATING

As we come to the end of our discussion about picky eating, I hope that I have empowered you to first, relax in the knowledge that you are not alone and that picky eating is normal and generally not something that will last forever. And second, I hope I have given you the knowledge and the tools to know how to respond to picky eating in a gentle way that will free both yourself and your toddler from some of the battles that can dominate mealtimes.

The most important part of feeding toddlers is building a framework around eating and mealtimes that enables us to focus less on the short-term meal-to-meal wins of "getting" our toddlers to eat and more on the long-term solutions that will help our kids to eat intuitively, laying the foundations for a having a lifelong good relationship with food. The truth is, when we're worried, we often lose sight of the bigger picture. Even when our toddlers are going through more challenging times with their eating, they are probably still getting most of what they need. If you find yourself second guessing your approach, adjust your expectations on how you view nutrient and food intake and think about what they are eating over the course of the week instead of meal to meal, or day to day.

Choking Hazard Guidelines (Ages 1-4)

As babies develop their eating skills and move through toddlerhood, we have more wiggle room when it comes to how we prepare and serve foods, so there are some choking hazard foods that we no longer have to modify at all (see below). With the eruption of molars, which are the primary teeth used for chewing and grinding down food, toddlers are able to manage more challenging textures, and the more advanced they become in their chewing skills, the more confident we feel at meal and snack times. This is great, but it's important to remember that we must continue to take special care with choking hazards and how we prepare and serve these foods to kids under four.

MINIMIZING THE RISK OF CHOKING

Safely preparing and serving foods is just one piece of the puzzle when it comes to reducing the risk of choking. The reality is, kids can choke on any food, so creating a safe eating environment is just as important as modifying choking hazards. Below I have put together my top tips for creating an eating environment that will allow your child to eat and explore foods as safely as possible.

- **CPR Course:** You may have already taken a pediatric first aid course when you introduced solids to your baby. If you haven't, I highly recommend taking one, so that you will know exactly what to do in the unlikely event that your child does choke.

- **Choking Hazards:** Be sure to modify all choking hazards before offering them to your child. Additionally, you should share this information with any caregivers that will be spending time with your child to ensure that they know how to safely prepare and serve foods, too.

- **Supervision:** It's easy to get distracted during mealtimes, but it's very important that a responsible adult is always present to supervise meals and snacks.

- **Movement and Posture:** Kids should be sitting or standing still when eating. Do not let your child walk, run, climb or jump when eating. Additionally, avoid offering your child food in their stroller or car seat. Also, where possible, ensure that your child is upright in a supportive chair, and never let your child eat while reclined or lying down.

- **Food Games:** Kids love to play, and making mealtimes fun is encouraged; however, refrain from playing risky food games that may involve your child throwing a piece food in the air and catching it with their mouth, even if that food is not considered a choking hazard.

- **Gagging:** Some toddlers may still gag from time to time. Gagging is not dangerous and does not indicate that your child is choking or is about to choke. If your toddler gags, do not panic and do not try to finger sweep the food out of their mouth, because you may accidently push the food into their windpipe. Instead, remain calm and wait patiently for the gag the pass.

- **Liquids:** Offer liquids alongside meals and snacks so that your child can wash down food as needed. For kids under two, you can offer water or milk (juice is not recommended); for kids over two, you can offer water, milk or an occasional small cup of watered-down fruit juice, if desired.

- **Take Time:** Allow plenty of time for your child to eat and enjoy their meal. Rushing kids can result in them trying to swallow food without chewing it properly. Additionally, young children are often in a hurry to leave the table so they can go and play, so be sure to remind them to slow down and chew their food properly.

- **New Foods:** Have your child try new foods at home before sending it to day care or school so that they can get used to new foods and textures in a familiar environment.

COMMON CHOKING HAZARDS FOR KIDS UNDER 4

Please note that the list below is not exhaustive. Please refer to current government guidelines for a comprehensive list.

CHOKING HAZARD	SAFE MODIFICATION
Chunks or spoonfuls of nut or seed butter	Spread thinly on foods, or stir into yogurt, oatmeal, or other pureed textures
String cheese or large chunks of hard cheese	Slice lengthways or chop into small bite-size pieces
Hot dogs and sausages	Slice into quarters lengthways, or chop into small bite-size pieces
Large chunks of meat or strips of tough, dry meat	Shred or cut into small bite-size pieces
Whole nuts and seeds	Finely chop or grind
Whole grapes and cherry/grape tomatoes	Quarter lengthwise
Whole strawberries	12–18 months: Sliced 18+ months: Whole or quartered if large, soft and ripe
Whole blueberries	12–24 months: Flatten into discs 24+ months: Halved, or whole if ripe and soft
Whole raspberries	Under 12 months: Cut in half or smush 12+ months: Whole if ripe and soft
Whole blackberries	12–24 months: Quartered lengthwise 24+ months: Whole if ripe and soft
Unripe pear	Steam or bake until soft
Clementine/satsuma segments	12–24 months: Remove fibrous spine and cut in half 24+ months: Halved with spine intact
Cherries	Remove pit and quarter lengthwise
Apple (raw)	12–24 months: Slice thinly or shred 24+ months: Slice thinly or serve whole
Baby carrots (raw)	12+ months: Cut into matchsticks or shred
Celery (raw)	12+ months: Slice thinly or cut into matchsticks
Olives	12+ months: Quarter lengthwise

Foods to Avoid Completely Until at Least Age 4:
- Whole kernel popcorn
- Hard chips, crisps and crackers
- Hard candy or sweets
- Marshmallows
- Chewing gum

Foods You No Longer Need to Modify (From 12 Months):
- Cooked peas can be served whole (no longer need to be flattened)
- Cooked corn kernels can be served whole (no longer need to be flattened)
- Soft fresh bread no longer needs to be toasted
- Apple and carrot can now be served raw if thinly sliced

How to Introduce & Manage Sugar in a Realistic Way

Introducing sugar to kids and managing sugar intake has become a hot topic over the years, and there is a lot of confusing, conflicting and often alarmist information out there that can make it difficult to know how to go about it in the best way. The fact is, sugar is everywhere, and for a vast majority of us, it's pretty much impossible to avoid. We know that we need to be mindful of sugar, but we also know that we need to be realistic in our approach because when we demonize and over-restrict sugar, we run the risk of creating the exact problems we are trying to avoid—which is a child that is obsessed with sweets!

In this chapter, I explore some of the ways we can help our kids to develop a healthy relationship with sugar using a gentle, low-stress approach. Your confidence will grow with the tools to manage their sugar intake while still prioritizing a varied diet and a healthy approach to food in general. Contrary to popular belief, these things can coexist, and it can be done without making sugar the main focus or something to fear!

WHEN TO INTRODUCE SUGAR

Kids Under 2 Years Old

For toddlers under 2 years old, it is recommended that we should avoid serving foods with added sugar. This includes natural sugars such as honey and maple syrup but does not include fruits and vegetables (pureed or otherwise), which are fine to use as sweeteners. Most babies and toddlers have a relatively small intake of food, and as such, we need to prioritize nutrient-dense foods in their diet so we can support them in meeting their nutritional needs. When sugar is present, it can reduce the intake of those nutrient-dense foods—so in other words, we need to make every bite count and sugar is not helpful in meeting that goal.

With that said, waiting until your toddler is 2 years old to introduce sugar may not be possible for many of us, and chances are your baby or toddler will have the occasional food with added sugar before then. This is okay! Putting huge amounts of pressure on yourself to ensure that your child doesn't have a single exposure to sugar before the age of 2 will only stand to serve your guilty conscience if you veer off course, and it won't support you and your child in developing and maintaining a healthy relationship with sugar overall.

What is more helpful is to take a more realistic approach and aim to manage sugar in a way that works best for your family and lifestyle, without guilt. Maybe you have older children that are enjoying some dessert at the table and your 1 year old notices, so you give them a few bites. Or maybe it's a special occasion or holiday and you want your child to try some of a traditional food your family loves. Or maybe you are unable to source a specific food you need without added sugar. Whatever the reason, it's okay to offer occasional bites of food with added sugar before they are two—it won't hurt them! Just be mindful of the foods you choose to serve regularly and keep their overall intake of sugar low, making food swaps whenever possible.

Kids Over 2 Years Old

Once your toddler turns 2 years old, you can begin to intentionally introduce foods with added sugars. Most toddlers are aware of sweets, cookies and desserts by now, but if your toddler is not, you don't have to introduce sugar right away and you can hold off for longer if you wish. But keep in mind that sugar is pretty much everywhere. Eventually, kids will be exposed to it, and if they haven't had it before, they may not know how to handle it, which could potentially lead to overeating and a preoccupation with sugary foods. We want our kids to develop and nurture a healthy relationship with all foods, including sugar, and the best way to achieve this is through exposure and by giving them opportunities to experience sugar and understand the way it makes them feel. So don't hold off too long!

HOW TO INTRODUCE & MANAGE SUGAR

Once you have decided to introduce sugar, you can do so with regularity. That doesn't mean you need to start offering it daily or going all out—it just means that you can include your toddler in enjoying desserts with the rest of the family in whatever way fits in with your routine. If your family set up is such that you never serve desserts, consider doing so occasionally and in a neutral way. I know that this can feel like an alien concept because sugar gets such a bad rap, but the research is clear in that the restriction of sugar only leads to kids wanting it more, and it is counterproductive to what we want to achieve in the long term. With this in mind, we want to ensure that our toddlers are getting at least some exposure so that they can learn how to manage sugar and see firsthand how it can be enjoyed as part of everyday life.

The main goal when introducing sugar is to be neutral and show our kids that it can be enjoyed as part of a balanced and nutritious diet and not something that is forbidden, to be feared or that they must restrict it in order to be healthy. And of course, it goes without saying that in general, we want to continue to be mindful of sugar and maintain our focus on offering a wide variety of foods. Even though it sounds counter-intuitive, by using sugar itself as a tool we can enable both ourselves and our kids to manage sugar intake, keeping sugar levels down overall.

How to Serve Desserts

When it comes to the business of actually offering sweets and desserts, it's best to treat them like any other food—this means bringing neutrality to the forefront, keeping the playing field level and being mindful of the language we use. Desserts and sweets are just that—desserts and sweets! Steer clear of calling them "treats" or labelling them as good or bad, or inferring that they are more or less satisfying than other foods. Just call them exactly what they are, without judgement.

We also want to avoid putting sweets and desserts on a pedestal by using them as a reward or bribe, and instead serve them *alongside* meals or snacks instead of afterwards. The latter is especially important as many kids may skip meals or snacks or eat past fullness (if completing part or all of the meal is a requirement for having dessert) in anticipation for dessert.

When you choose to serve dessert (which doesn't have to be every day), serve it on the table as part of the family meal or snack or directly on your toddler's plate with the rest of their food, and although this may seem crazy, always allow your toddler to choose *when* to eat the dessert. If they choose to eat it first, resist the urge to discourage this—just continue to eat your own meal and allow your toddler to explore and handle it themselves. You'll be surprised to see that with consistency in this approach, your toddler will likely eat the other foods on their plate, as well as the dessert. If you find this approach challenging and feel that your toddler is preoccupied with dessert foods, there are ways that you can introduce boundaries that don't emphasise restriction, which I talk about in the Finding a Balance section (page 20) of this chapter.

If your toddler is used to having dessert served after a meal, this will be somewhat of a novelty to start and it's likely that at first, they may only eat the dessert and decide not to eat anything else. As hard as this is to allow, it's important to hold the boundary and stay neutral—it takes time (sometimes a long time) to unlearn habits, and your toddler will likely test this boundary by seeing if you are *really* serious about your new approach. Over time they will adjust and will begin enjoying other foods alongside dessert.

I also want to add here that it is okay to serve sweets and dessert foods outside of meals and snacks on occasion. Maybe you are on a family outing and want to enjoy an ice cream, or maybe you are visiting friends who have prepared a delicious cake to share—whatever the situation, it's okay to be flexible and realistic in your approach, which will further drive the point home that sweets are just another food and not something to be singled out and stressed about.

Finding a Balance

You're probably wondering how much dessert you should serve in one sitting and what you should do if your toddler requests seconds or thirds, and how you can strike a balance that allows them to explore and manage sugar on their own terms, but within reason, that isn't restriction. There are two ways you can approach this—first, you can choose to offer your toddler as much dessert as they want in the moment and allow them to figure out how it makes them feel. It's likely that at first, they will eat too much, but this will give you an opportunity to open up an age-appropriate conversation about what they are feeling physically. This doesn't mean focusing on the negative—we still want to keep that neutrality going, but you can encourage them to make that connection and develop an understanding about how their bodies feel when they eat more than they can handle. Developing this understanding is a process that involves lots of trial and error and the only way for them to figure it out is to practice!

If you decide to take this approach, you'll have to dig deep and resist the urge to cut them off from their sugar intake mid meal and trust them to figure out how to self-regulate how much they should eat—it may not happen on the first go, but they will get there with practice!

The second approach is to offer a set amount of dessert that you have decided *prior* to a meal or snack and stick within that boundary. If you want to provide just one serving, that's okay—just be sure that the serving is reasonable, and you aren't offering deliberately small portions that could make your child feel restricted. If your toddler requests more dessert, you can explain using neutral and age-appropriate language that this is all we have for dessert at this time, and there will be other opportunities to eat these foods again and redirect back to their meal if they are still hungry. The goal with this explanation is to make sure they know that desserts will be featured again, so they don't need to become preoccupied with "getting" more or become worried that there will be a lengthy wait until the next offering.

If you choose to take this approach, you should still find ways for your child to have occasional opportunities to eat unlimited amounts of these foods, so they can learn their limits, tune into their body and develop an understanding of how these foods make them feel. One way I like to do this with my own toddler is to offer unlimited amounts of his favorite ice cream every Saturday. At first, he ate several servings, but it didn't take long for this to reduce—then he surprised me one random Saturday by refusing ice cream altogether and requesting cheese and crackers instead!

Whichever method you choose, remember that you are the parent, so you get to decide *what* the dessert is and *when* to serve it. They also don't always have to be rich, high-sugar foods—you can alternate and serve both light and indulgent desserts, and you can absolutely incorporate nutrition into them. My kids love it when I serve strawberries, cream and a drizzle of maple syrup for dessert! Likewise, you don't have to serve dessert every day. If 2 to 3 times per week is what your family prefers, then that's perfectly fine. Striking a balance is going to look different for everyone, and it may take some trial and error before you find your sweet spot.

Lastly, it is completely normal for kids to enjoy desserts—they taste nice, and you will most definitely get requests for them when they aren't available. This doesn't mean that your toddler is sweet obsessed or that we need to discourage them from having preferences in a quest to dull their cravings. Our main goal is to support our kids in learning how to regulate their sugar intake through exposure and without demonizing sugar and unintentionally creating an environment where desserts become a shiny and unattainable treat. Not everything we eat must serve a nutritional or health goal. It's okay to eat foods just because we enjoy them and they bring us together as a family to create happy memories together—all foods can fit into a balanced and nutritious diet!

Age Suitability & Portion Size

AGE SUITABILITY

The majority of the recipes in this book are suitable from 6 months old (modified accordingly). Some recipes contain natural added sugars, which can usually be omitted for toddlers under 2 years old—those that can't have been labelled as "Age Suitability: 2+ years." However, a few bites here and there for toddlers under 2 won't hurt. Please note that any recipes containing honey are not suitable for kids under one due to the risk of infant botulism.

PORTION SIZE

Portion sizes shown in this book are for guidance only. Some kids will eat more or less than this, and that is okay. I recommend starting with small portions and topping up as needed.

Common Questions

CAN I STILL BREASTFEED MY TODDLER?

Absolutely! The nutritional benefits of breastfeeding continue long after infancy, and the World Health Organization (WHO) recommends breastfeeding until 2 years of age, or longer if you and your child want to. If your toddler is breastfeeding three to four times per day, you do not need to offer cow's milk or other milks as a drink.

MY TODDLER DRINKS COW/PLANT-BASED MILK. HOW MUCH MILK DO THEY NEED AND WHEN SHOULD IT BE SERVED?

Cow's milk and nutritionally appropriate plant-based milks are a convenient source of calories, fat, protein and calcium for growing toddlers. However, milk is *complementary* to food, and as such, drinking too much milk can crowd out the other foods and nutrients that toddlers need.

Current recommendations are that toddlers should have no more than 16 ounces (480 ml) of cow's milk or plant-based milk per day, because drinking more than this can result in a decreased appetite for solid foods and has been associated with an increased risk of iron deficiency. To help keep milk intake within these parameters, aim to serve milk as part of a meal or snack (except for bedtime milk, if applicable). And don't forget that the milk you add to cereal and other foods/recipes counts as part of their daily intake. While a little more milk (than recommended) here and there is not an issue, it helps to be mindful of this when adding up their intake for the day.

MY TODDLER WON'T DRINK MILK. WHAT SHOULD I DO?

If your toddler doesn't like to drink milk, or drinks very little milk, you don't need to worry! Yes, milk is a convenient source of calories, fat, protein and calcium, but toddlers don't actually *need* milk to thrive. There are many other ways for them to get these nutrients from other foods.

For example, below is a list of just some (not all) of the foods that are rich in all four of the nutrients mentioned above:

- Cheese
- Yogurt
- Almond butter
- Baked beans
- Canned salmon
- Chia seeds

The main thing to remember is that exposing toddlers to a wide variety of foods is going to be far more helpful to them in meeting their overall nutritional needs than any one food will ever be, so consistency in this approach is key. With that said, if you feel that your toddler would benefit from having at least some level of milk intake, you can incorporate it into their diet in other ways, such as adding it to smoothies, milkshakes, oatmeal, white sauces, rice puddings, etc., but never hide the fact that these foods contain milk. If they ask, be honest!

MY TODDLER STILL EATS WITH THEIR HANDS. HOW CAN I ENCOURAGE THEM TO USE CUTLERY?

For toddlers, using their hands is the quickest and most efficient way for them to get food into their tummies, and for many, this is all they really care about. What's more, toddlers enjoy touching and feeling the different textures and temperatures of foods, and it is great for sensory exploration. This is an important part of learning how to eat. Learning how to use cutlery will naturally follow on from this. Some kids will enter toddlerhood already using cutlery, whereas others don't start working on it until closer to 2 or even 3 years old. All of this is completely normal and developmentally appropriate, and if your toddler is taking their time to learn this skill, it's not something you need to worry about or that needs to be rushed. With all this said, there are some ways that you can gently encourage and support your toddler in learning this skill. See the following list for some ideas.

Tips to get kids to use cutlery:

- **Use Kids' Cutlery:** Adult cutlery tends to have longer handles that can be tricky for toddlers to use, and the fork or spoon bowl may be too big to fit in their mouths. Instead, offer smaller-sized toddler-friendly cutlery that they can comfortably fit in their hands and mouth.
- **Modelling:** Toddlers are natural copycats, so without a doubt, the best way to teach them how to use cutlery is to let them see you using yours! Be sure to create plenty of opportunities to eat meals together as a family so your toddler can see how it's done.
- **Exposure and Consistency:** Provide your toddler with cutlery at every meal, even if they ignore it. Although preloading spoons is more commonly associated with introducing solids, it can be very useful for your toddler too. You can preload their spoon or fork at the start of the meal and simply place it on their plate. They may well discard the cutlery after they eat the single bite of food, but doing so consistently will help them to connect the dots over time.
- **Demonstrate:** Some toddlers may benefit from a physical, hands-on demonstration on how to use the correct motion of their wrists to scoop foods or their fingers to grasp and gently stab and pick up food with a fork. If your toddler is happy to let you do so, you can place your hand over theirs while they are holding cutlery and show them the correct motion—but only do this once or twice, then let them practice for the rest of the meal themselves, if they want to do so. Some toddlers may not like this, and if this is the case, don't push it. Simply leave them to eat their meal as they wish.
- **Patience:** There is no rush when it comes to using cutlery. There is wide scope for what is developmentally normal and often all that is needed is to be patient and give your toddler some time.

DIVIDED OR OPEN PLATES—WHICH IS BEST?

There's a lot of debate over which type of plate is best for babies and toddlers, and it typically boils down to divided plates vs. open plates. If you are only planning on having one plate for your toddler, then a regular, non-divided plate would be the best option. It will grow with your toddler and last longer, and it's what they will be expected to use more widely in their day-to-day lives, such as at restaurants or when visiting friends and family.

However, there are benefits to using divided plates too—I personally like that I can incorporate several elements of a meal into one plate that would otherwise have to be separated (such as grilled cheese and soup) without having to use separate tableware. Divided plates tend to have higher walls, which mean less mess. They can also be a great option for picky eaters who do not like their food to touch. With this in mind, I do recommend having one of each for the sake of convenience and variety, but whatever works best for your toddler and your lifestyle is perfectly fine, including using divided plates exclusively.

You may have heard that introducing divided plates from a young age and using them exclusively will encourage or increase picky eating, as they introduce and carry forward the concept of separating foods, but there is no evidence to support this theory. And in any case, the perceived "risk" is easily remedied by simply mixing different foods in the same sections of the plate (such as curry and rice), which is something I have always done when using divided plates with my children.

HOW LONG CAN MY TODDLER USE A HIGH CHAIR?

A comfortable high chair that supports your toddler in sitting in the correct position can be the key to successful mealtimes, and it is recommended that they continue to use a high chair for as long as is feasibly possible. What's more, eating in a suitable high chair encourages safe eating habits and keeps their mess more contained. Once you transition your toddler to a booster seat or a suitable dining chair, it might be hard to go back—so be sure before making your decision!

Signs Your Toddler Is Ready to Transition to a Booster Seat or Regular Chair

Comfortability of High Chair

When it comes to deciding whether or not to transition your toddler to a booster seat or suitable dining chair, the first thing to consider is the style and comfortability of their high chair and if it ensures the following:

- It is still spacious enough for your toddler to sit in comfortably, and they can freely move their arms to rest their elbows on the table or tray.
- It has an adjustable footrest that provides stability and ensures that your toddler's knees are at a 90-degree angle.
- The seat doesn't slouch backwards and allows your toddler to sit with their hips at a 90-degree angle.

If your toddler's high chair meets **all** three of these requirements, then they can continue to use it during meal and snack times. If not, then it is time to transition to a booster seat or a suitable toddler-friendly dining chair. It is also recommended that toddlers should be brought up to the table for meal times as soon as possible, so if their high chair tray is not removable, you may consider transitioning, but it's perfectly fine to wait until you feel that your toddler is ready.

Your Toddler No Longer Likes to Sit in Their High Chair

If your toddler becomes upset or disruptive when placed in their high chair, it could be that they simply no longer like sitting in their high chair and would prefer to sit on a chair like everyone else. If you are still using a tray, then consider removing this and pulling your toddler's high chair up to the table before transitioning—sometimes this is enough to solve the problem.

Your Toddler Is Able to Climb Out of Their High Chair

Once your toddler can wriggle out of their harness and climb out of the high chair, it is no longer safe to use it, and it's time to make the transition. If your toddler is just a spontaneous daredevil and doesn't mind sitting in their high chair for the most part, you may consider switching out the harness to something they can't wriggle out of, but depending on their age, this may not be worth the expense for just a few extra weeks or months of high chair use.

MY TODDLER THROWS FOOD, WHAT CAN I DO?

One of the most frustrating aspects of feeding babies and toddlers is food throwing! Not only does it create even more mess for us to clean, but it also creates food waste, which can be a real problem for many of us.

There are many reasons why toddlers throw food. Following are some common reasons.

Not Hungry or Finished Their Meal

When toddlers are no longer hungry, they might communicate this by throwing their food. You can get ahead of this by only serving small portions to start, and then topping off their plates as needed. This way, if they do throw their food, it will only be a small amount. Additionally, clear your toddler's plate once you are sure they are finished eating, and if you still want them to sit at the table, you can offer a toy or activity to keep them occupied.

Challenging Foods

Sometimes, toddlers throw foods that they are not sure about or that they find challenging to eat. Maybe it's a new food, or a food they are finding it difficult to self-feed—for example, they may struggle to eat a smooth soup from a spoon and would find it easier to drink it from a cup, or maybe they would prefer to eat a deconstructed burger as they find it tricky to handle one that is fully assembled. You might not always figure out the answer, but it's something worth thinking about.

Pressured to Eat

Toddlers don't like to feel pressured to eat, and it can quickly descend into food throwing. Aim to keep mealtimes stress free by taking the focus off of the food (including positive reinforcement for eating) and instead shift the focus on spending quality time together.

Boredom

Toddlers just want to enjoy themselves and to them, throwing food is fun. This often happens when they have been sitting at the table too long (for them) and are keen to get down and play.

Attention Seeking and Testing Boundaries

Whether it's positive or negative, toddlers like all types of attention. Testing boundaries in their day-to-day lives is a normal part of their development. Believe it or not, it's how they nurture relationships and form bonds with their caregivers.

Food-Throwing Solutions

My main strategy for dealing with food throwing is redirection, which simply means to shift the focus of my toddler's attention to engaging in preferred behavior. If I tell my toddler not to throw food, he typically responds by looking me in the eye and throwing more food, which would in turn make me even more frustrated. What I find more effective is to encourage the preferred behavior I want by saying "food stays on the plate." Now that he has a deeper level of understanding, I often provide a "no thank you bowl" and encourage him to put the food he doesn't want in the bowl so he doesn't have to have it on his plate if that's his preference. Telling toddlers what they *can* do often generates better results than telling them what they can't do.

Of course, redirection doesn't always work, and when this happens, I ignore the food throwing entirely. That means putting on my best poker face and not reacting in any way when he throws food—this includes picking the food up off the floor when he throws it, which he often considers a game. This approach worked very well when he was younger, as he had a shorter attention span and would quickly lose interest and start doing something else. As frustrating as it is, food throwing does not last forever and eventually toddlers do grow out of it, so if you are currently going through it, hang in there and this too shall pass!

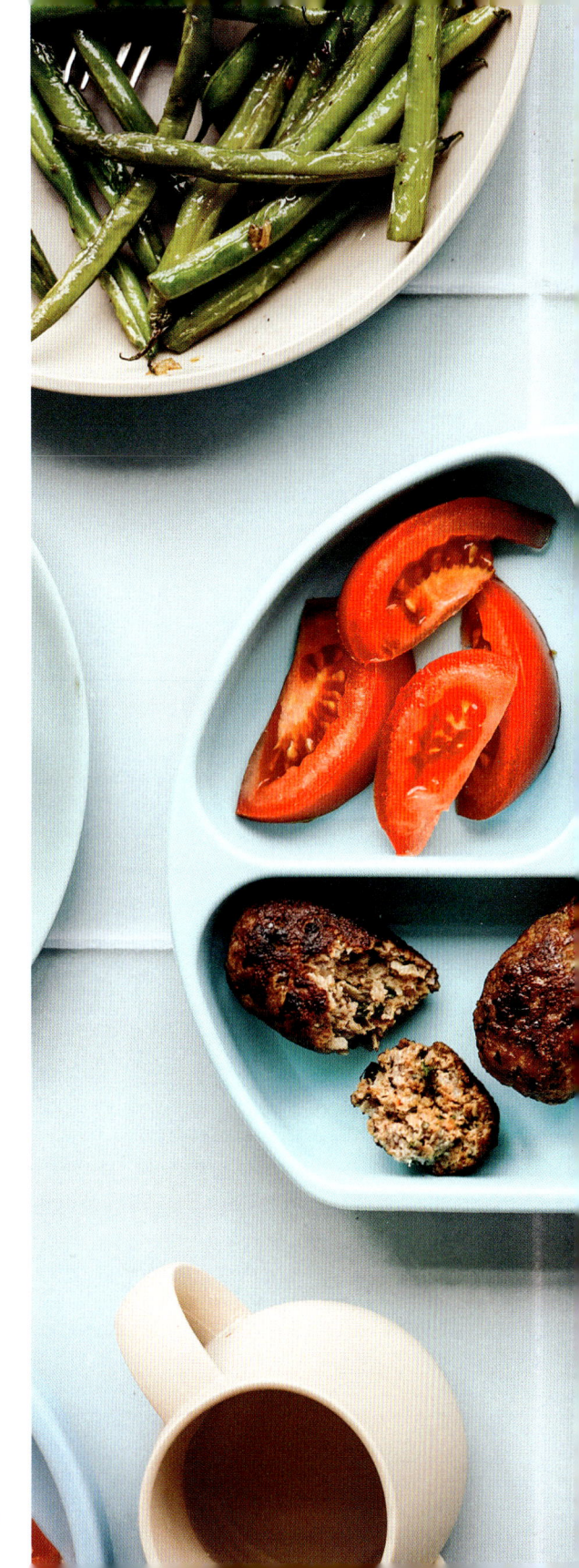

CHAPTER 2

Smart Snacking

I am so excited about including this chapter in this book because the topic of snacks is something I am constantly asked about on my Instagram page. From what I've heard, and from my own personal experience as a mom of five, introducing snacks can feel like an overwhelming prospect when we have just gotten the hang of providing three meals a day. On one hand, we want to put in the effort to make sure our children are eating as well as possible and that we are offering them a variety of nutritious and tasty foods. But on the other hand, we have limited time and energy to pull it all together, and then of course there is the simultaneous challenge of parenting an independent toddler who is developing their own tastes and preferences, not just gobbling everything up as they might have done as babies. It's a lot to juggle, and it can feel like a huge mountain to climb!

But I am here to give you a hand. In this chapter, I walk you through my no-nonsense, stress-free approach to snacks that will work *with* you and your toddler, and not against! I will also share my tried and tested top tips and ideas for easy, balanced and delicious snacks that won't leave you feeling burnt out and overstretched.

Introducing Snacks

Once your baby turns one, it's time to think about introducing snacks. You're probably wondering how on earth you're going to fit in yet more time in the kitchen, but don't worry! When snacks are done smartly, they are not a big deal, and with a little forethought, snack time will be an invaluable part of your child's day. Now, I do want to highlight here that not *all* toddlers are ready for snacks the very moment they turn one—or it may be the case that they only need one snack for a while, or maybe two very light snacks, or just a bedtime snack, etc. I like to look at introducing snacks as a transition, and like all transitions, some kids are ready to jump in head first, while others may dip their toes in initially and need some time to adjust to get to where they *personally* need to be.

WHY SNACKS ARE IMPORTANT

Most kids love snacks, and many would happily eat them all day and skip their main meals altogether. But while snacks can be massively appealing to kids (and perhaps not always for the best of reasons), snacks are actually crucial in two key ways:

1. Snacks keep our kids going between meals. Toddlers have high energy needs, and coupled with having small tummies, they burn through the foods they eat quickly, so it's important that they have an opportunity to fuel up and maintain their energy levels every 2 to 3 hours.

2. Snacks are essential for filling in nutritional gaps, especially for kids who may not eat much at mealtimes. Kids have demanding nutritional needs, but they also have ever-changing appetites—they may eat very little at one meal or snack, and then a ton of food at another, or even just small amounts at every meal and snack. If they don't eat much in one sitting, having the opportunity to eat again in a few hours means they will not have to rely on limited eating windows to meet their nutritional needs.

Healthy Snacks for Toddlers & Kids

WHAT IS CONSIDERED A NUTRITIOUS SNACK FOR KIDS?

For many kids, the most appealing snacks are the ones that I refer to as crinkly bag snacks. They are usually simple carbs, such as crackers, dried cereal, crisps/chips and so on. Now, while these foods are very convenient and absolutely *can* be a part of a nutritious snack, they are often low in fat and protein, something that kids need to feel full and to sustain them until the next meal. Also, it's often the case that we reserve these foods for snack time only, which creates the idea that they are special, or perhaps a treat. What tends to happen as a result of this is that kids will happily eat less of a meal you have prepared in anticipation of a specific type of "snack" food they have become accustomed to, and they may become preoccupied with these snack foods and ask for them constantly throughout the day.

When thinking about offering nutritious snacks, its more useful to think of *all* types of foods as snack food options, and in turn, incorporate the crinkly bag snacks into your kids' main meals too. This levels out the playing field and sends a clear message to kids that there is no hierarchy when it comes to food, they can enjoy all foods together, and there is no need to "hold out" for snack time or for a specific type of food.

MINI MEALS AS SNACKS

Shifting your mindset from snack foods to mini meals is a game changer. Now don't panic! This doesn't mean you will need to create six main meals a day! Mini meals are simply snacks that mimic small meals in the sense that they are made up of 2 to 3 food groups, but they are still quick and easy! For example, instead of serving cheese-flavored crackers as a snack, you could serve plain crackers with sliced or soft cheese and a piece of fruit on the side. Mini meals do not require a ton of work, and you can still rely on convenient, quick, easy-to-prep foods to create balanced mini meal snacks for your toddler.

Thinking of snacks as mini meals means that kids are exposed to more variety over the course of the day, and it allows for the fact that kids can often be hungrier at snack times. Providing a balanced mini meal snack makes the most of these hungry windows and makes it more likely that they will be satisfied between meals.

Simple Snack Building Formula

Balancing snacks is easy! All you need to do is include the following:

High Protein Food and/or Source of Fat
Foods that are high in protein and healthy fats are crucial for keeping kids feeling full. While carbs are important and do provide energy, kids burn through them very fast and are left feeling hungry again soon after. Offering a source of protein and/or fat as part of a snack helps kids to fill that gap and keep them going until the next meal.

Fruit and/or Veggie
Fruits and vegetables are a great source of fiber, and fiber also contributes to helping kids feel full. Additionally, including fruits and veggies as part of a snack helps to expose kids to more variety throughout the day and helps to support them in meeting their nutritional needs over time. You can find examples of simple mini meal snacks in the "Easy Balanced Snack Examples" section on page 30.

WHAT ABOUT CARBS?
You may be wondering why carbohydrates aren't listed as an essential snack component in this snack balancing formula. After all, kids *do* need carbs for energy, and it is **not** recommended to limit them. Well, many high protein and high fat foods have carbohydrates, as do many fruits and vegetables, so by following this snack building formula, your child will be getting carbs too. But you absolutely can beef up the carb content of a snack if you wish to do so—just be sure to include a variety of carbs throughout the day, including whole grains, so that your little one will get the most staying power from their snacks.

Scheduling Snacks

SHOULD WE SCHEDULE SNACKS?
I've already talked about the importance of food schedules for kids, and snacks are no exception to this. One way that you can pretty much guarantee that your toddler won't eat much at mealtimes is to let them snack as often as they want or graze all day. It's important that we give kids enough time to build up an appetite so that they come to the table hungry, and scheduling snacks will support them in this.

How you work snacks into your feeding routine will depend on your child and your personal circumstances, and you may need to play around with timings at first until you find your sweet spot. A great starting point is to plan snacks midway between meals or at the very least avoid serving snacks too close to meals.

HOW MANY SNACKS SHOULD KIDS HAVE?
Depending on your child's age and eating habits, two to three snacks a day is the general rule of thumb. Younger toddlers may take some time to build up to two or three snacks, and many kids will not even need the third (bedtime) snack at all. All kids have differing appetites. Some children are able to pack in a lot of food at mealtimes and will only need one snack, or possibly no snacks at all. This is okay too, and children should never be encouraged to eat more food than their bodies are telling them that they need. Just be mindful that a child's fueling needs can change over time or even quite quickly, so you should continue to offer them the option of a snack (or snacks) just in case they decide they need more food after all.

SHOULD YOU OFFER A BEDTIME SNACK?

Bedtime snacks can be a super helpful way to ensure that kids have had enough to eat, and they can be a familiar part of their bedtime routine, but not all kids need or want them. You might consider offering a bedtime snack if your child hasn't eaten much of their evening meal and you don't want them to go to bed hungry. If they did eat their dinner, but bedtime is not for another couple of hours, or you just feel that your child would benefit from having another opportunity to eat and get in some extra nutrients and calories, then it's worth offering a bedtime snack. You know your child best!

While bedtime snacks can be a great addition to your child's eating routine, they shouldn't be exciting; in fact, they should be boring! If your child anticipates that their bedtime snack will be a food that they really love or some kind of treat, then they may be tempted to eat less of their dinner and hold out for that alluring bedtime snack. Keep the foods simple and varied and set the scene as just another time to eat.

Tips for Stress-Free Snack Times

PLAN AHEAD

Snack time can creep up on you, and you don't want to get caught out on a limb! Take some time at the start of the week to plan out snacks and be sure to include all the items you will need on your grocery list. You don't need to assign specific snacks to specific times or days but having some preplanned balanced snack combos in mind will help you avoid any last-minute fumbling in the cupboard!

BATCH COOK

I am a huge advocate of batch cooking, and I always try to keep a selection of foods in the freezer that I can defrost ahead of time or in the microwave for quick, tasty and nutritious snacks. You can find some freezer-friendly batch-cook snack options in Chapter 6 (page 129), but remember, all foods can be snack foods, so don't limit your options. If you want to serve a pancake or a waffle for a snack or use up your leftovers from lunch or dinner, then go for it!

FOOD PREP

Prepping fruits and veggies ahead of time is also a great time saver. You can wash, peel and prep fruits and veggies at the beginning of the week and store them in easy access tubs in the refrigerator. For grab-and-go options, prep single servings and store them in small airtight containers that can be thrown into your changing bag on the way out the door. Not only is this convenient and time saving, but your family will also likely eat more fruits and veggies as a result.

BE FLEXIBLE

For the most part, we need to be consistent in not serving food outside of our schedule. However, there are times when we need to allow some flexibility. For instance, your child may have had an especially active day and would benefit from having a scheduled snack brought forward or even an additional snack altogether. It's okay to be flexible when needed and adjust your approach depending on what's happening at the time.

MANAGE SNACK OBSESSED KIDS

It's not unusual for kids to become snack obsessed, and it typically occurs when kids have gotten used to having certain types of foods as snacks. One way you can work through this is to regularly serve the foods you have reserved for snack time in their main meals and be sure to include "meal" foods in their snacks. Blurring the lines between what they consider to be snack vs. meal foods helps kids to stop obsessing over a particular food they want and learn that all foods can be enjoyed together.

BE KIND TO YOURSELF! CONSISTENCY IS KEY, BUT PERFECTION IS IMPOSSIBLE.

This is my mantra when it comes to all areas of feeding my kids. Striving for perfection is an unrealistic and unattainable goal that will leave you feeling burnt out and exhausted! Sometimes we are unable to stick to our meal and snack schedule. Sometimes it's just crackers for a snack because that's all that we can manage in that particular moment. I try my best to be consistent with my approach, but I never feel guilty for veering off course, and neither should you. We are all human, and a scattering of unbalanced or unscheduled snacks are not going to undo your hard work or cause any long-lasting effects to your child. The less we stress about eating perfectly, and the more we allow ourselves the grace to just eat and enjoy the foods we love, the much happier and healthier we will be!

Easy Balanced Snack Examples

The first snack list includes examples of quick, balanced snacks that are easy "throw together" snacks, and the second list features easy balanced snacks that are included in this cookbook. I recommend batch cooking the recipes listed in advance and storing them in your refrigerator or freezer so that you can pull these snacks together in mere minutes, as needed!

QUICK & EASY "THROW TOGETHER" SNACKS

1. Whole-grain crackers and cheese + strawberries
2. Yogurt with hulled hemp hearts + fresh mango chunks
3. Hummus + sliced bell pepper
4. Sliced banana and thinly spread nut or seed butter
5. Cottage cheese + red grapes
6. Smoothie or smoothie popsicle
7. Mashed avocado on rice cake + hulled hemp hearts
8. Nut or seed butter toast + apple
9. Applesauce + finely chopped or ground nuts and seeds
10. Pancakes + mashed fruit + chia seeds
11. Hardboiled egg + green peas
12. Full-fat milk or nondairy milk of choice + banana
13. Kefir + clementine
14. Granola bar + sliced pear
15. Milk + fruit and nut/seed bar

BALANCED SNACKS USING THE RECIPES IN THIS BOOK

1. Orange & Raspberry Muffin (page 131) + milk
2. Apple & Carrot Snack Bar (page 145) + fresh pineapple
3. No-Bake Multigrain Cereal Bar (page 132) + fruit cup
4. Easy Peachy Smoothie Bowl Popsicle (page 46) + granola bar
5. Iron-Rich Almond & Coconut Cookie (page 138) + banana
6. Cheesy Broccoli Balls (page 142) + fresh salsa dip
7. Toddler-Friendly Nut-Free Granola (page 38) + yogurt
8. Lemon & Blueberry Yogurt Muffin (page 146)
9. Whole-Wheat Protein Blender Waffle (page 37) + unsweetened applesauce
10. Iron-Rich Almond & Coconut Cookie (page 138) + milk + fresh raspberries
11. Bite-Size Fruity Cheesecake Strudel (page 135)
12. Pumpkin Pie Mini Muffin (page 141) + yogurt
13. Avocado Egg Salad (page 94) + whole grain crackers
14. Crispy Sweet Corn Fritters (page 98) + Homemade Marinara Dipping Sauce (page 127)
15. Chocolate Oat Bites (page 149) + clementine

Speedy Snack Cheat Sheet

Here is a rundown of some foods you can create balanced snacks from, categorized by food group for your ease. This list is not extensive, but just something for you to reference when you need some inspiration. Veggies can sometimes be tricky because many of them need to be cooked first, and in these cases I tend to fall back on leftover veggies from previous meals. Also, remember to prep and portion out your fruits and veggies at the beginning of the week to save time, and always keep a few options of prebaked muffins, waffles and pancakes in the freezer to beef up the carb content of your snacks, if desired.

PROTEIN	FAT	GRAINS (OPTIONAL)	FRUIT	VEGETABLES
Nut butters: • Peanut • Almond • Cashew Nuts, chopped or ground: • Peanuts • Almonds • Cashews • Hazelnuts • Pistachio nuts • Walnuts Seed butters: • Sunflower • Pumpkin • Hemp Seeds, chopped or ground: • Chia (whole) • Hulled hemp • Flaxseed • Sunflower • Pumpkin • Sesame Soya butter Full-fat cow's milk Nondairy milk: • Soy • Pea Full-fat Greek yogurt, kefir or natural yogurt	Nut butters: • Peanut • Almond • Cashew Nuts, chopped or ground: • Peanuts • Almonds • Cashews • Hazelnuts • Pistachio nuts • Walnuts Seed butters: • Sunflower • Pumpkin • Hemp Seeds, chopped or ground: • Chia (whole) • Hulled hemp • Flaxseed • Sunflower • Pumpkin • Sesame Soya butter Full-fat cow's milk Nondairy milk: • Soy • Pea Full-fat Greek yogurt, kefir or natural yogurt	Bread, fresh or toasted: • Whole grain • Sprouted • Bread rolls • Bagels • Pita • Naan English muffins and tortilla wraps Fruit bread and hot cross buns Crackers and breadsticks Rice cakes Dry cereal, such as multigrain hoops Oat and cereal bars (see Chapter 6 [page 129]) Store-bought bars: • Larabar™ • think!® bar • N'eat® bar Veggie sticks or baked pea snacks Muffins (see Chapter 6 [page 129])	Apple, applesauce, apple chips Apricots, fresh or dried Avocado and guacamole Banana and plantain Blackberries Blueberries Cherries, pips removed Citrus: • Oranges • Clementine • Satsumas • Grapefruit Dried fruit: • Apricots • Dates • Raisins Figs Fruit cups (in juice) Fruit juice	Avocado Beets Bell peppers Broccoli (leftovers) Brussels sprouts (leftovers) Carrots, raw (shredded or cut into matchsticks) or leftovers Cauliflower, leftovers Celery, cut into matchsticks Cherry or grape tomatoes, quartered Cucumber Dips: • Guacamole • Mild fresh salsa Edamame Eggplant, leftovers (see page 123) Green peas, cooked from frozen or canned

(Continued)

PROTEIN	FAT	GRAINS (OPTIONAL)	FRUIT	VEGETABLES
Full-fat kefir	Full-fat kefir	Waffles and pancakes (see Chapter 3 on page 35)	Freeze-dried fruit	Jicama
Full-fat cheese: · Hard cheese · Mozzarella · Cream cheese · Cottage cheese	Full-fat cheese: · Hard cheese · Mozzarella · Cream cheese · Cottage cheese	Chickpea and lentil pasta Noodles	Grapes, quartered Kiwi	Kale chips Lettuce Mushrooms, leftovers
Egg: · Hard boiled · Egg salad (page 94)	Butter Egg: · Hard boiled · Egg salad (page 94)		Mango, fresh or dried Melon: · Cantaloupe · Honey dew · Watermelon	Olives, pitted and quartered Parsnips, leftovers Pickles
Nitrate-free deli meats: · Turkey · Chicken · Ham/pork · Beef	Dips: · Lemon Garlic Dip (page 116) · Hummus · Guacamole · Mayonnaise · Ranch		Papaya Passion fruit	Plantain chips Potatoes, leftovers
Smoked sausage			Peaches and nectarines	Roasted seaweed
Canned fish: · Tuna · Salmon · Sardines	Oils: · Olive · Avocado · Coconut		Pear, ripe Persimmon	Sauerkraut Sugar snap and snow peas
Smoked salmon			Pineapple	Sweet corn, cooked from frozen or canned
Tofu and tempeh	Coconut: · Shredded or desiccated · Coconut yogurt · Whipped coconut cream		Plum Pomegranate	Sweet potatoes, leftovers
Dips: · Lemon Garlic Dip (page 116) · Hummus · Mayonnaise			Raspberries	Tomato, regular and sun dried
Beans, canned: · Chickpea · Cannellini · Kidney · Butter bean	Chocolate Oat Bites (page 149)		Strawberries Tomato	Zucchini, raw (cut into matchsticks) or leftovers
Chickpea puffs				
Oats: · Oatmeal · Granola (page 38) · Oat bar (page 145) · Oat cake cups (page 50)				
Chocolate Oat Bites (page 149)				

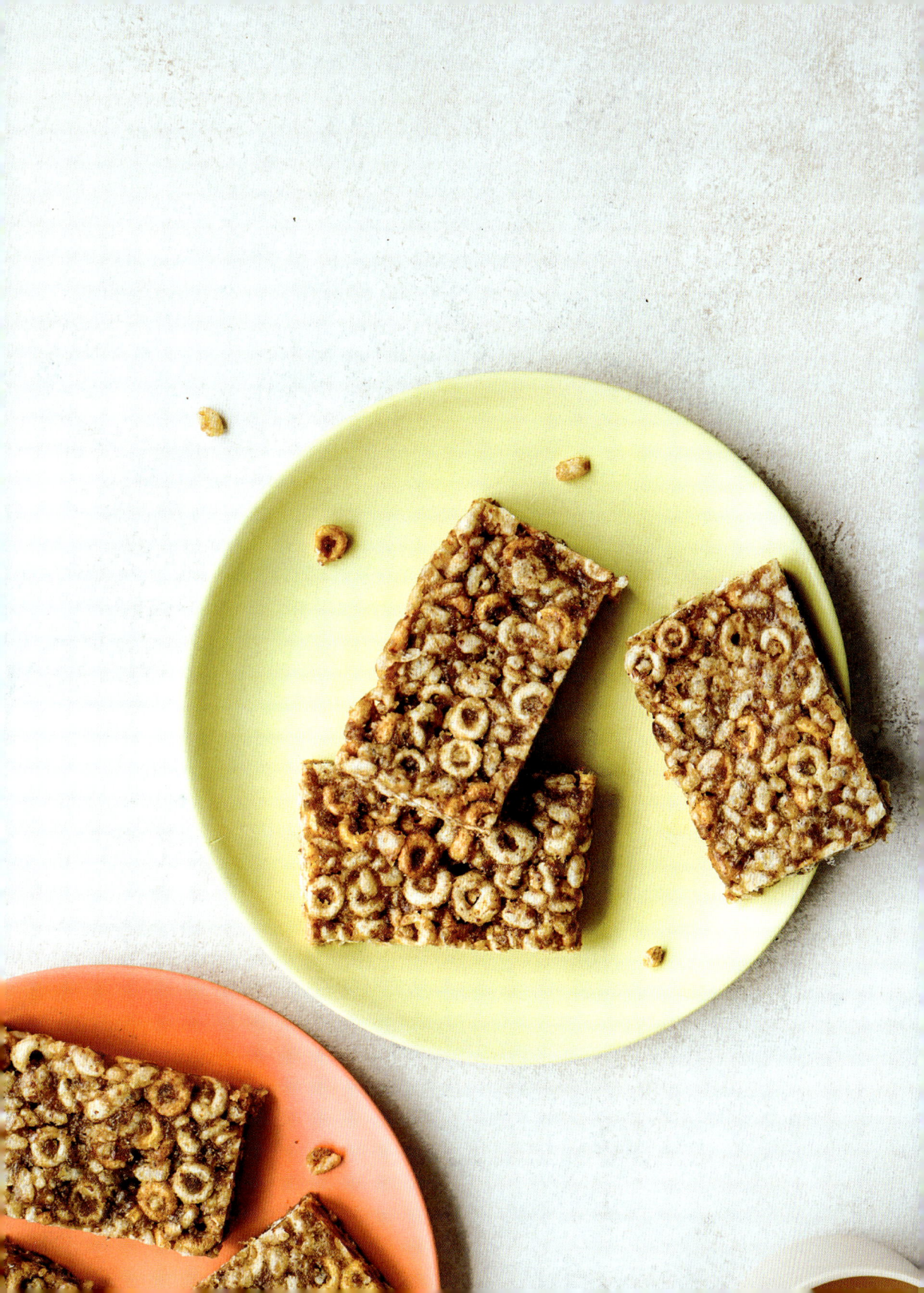

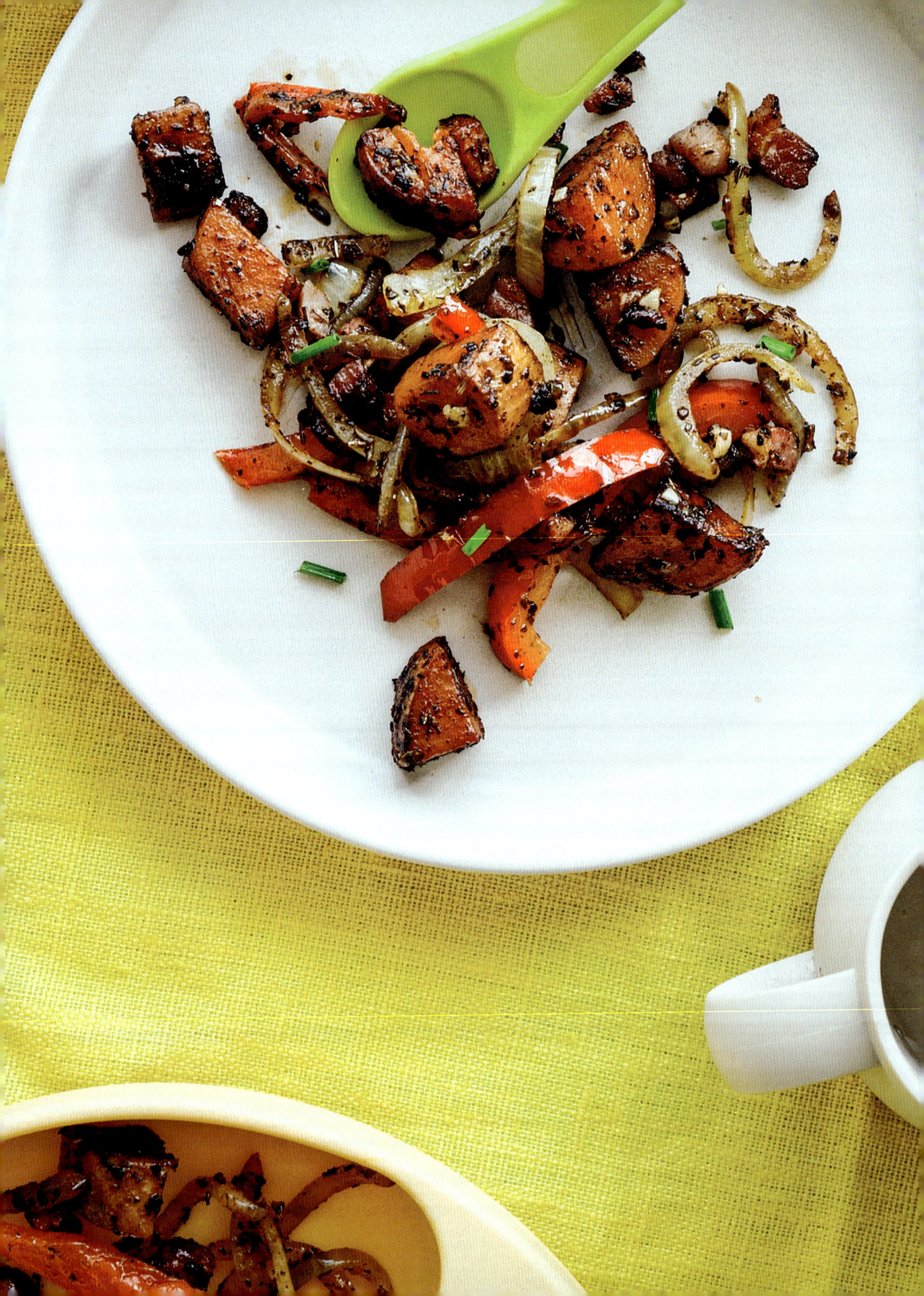

CHAPTER 3

Making the Most of Breakfast

Let's get your family off to a great start to the day with this selection of mouthwatering breakfast recipes that will also get your toddler excited about coming to the table! Almost all of the recipes can be made ahead of time for simple and fuss-free breakfasts on those super busy mornings.

Please note that many of the recipes in Chapter 6: Make-Ahead Snacks & Bakes (page 129) can be served for breakfast too!

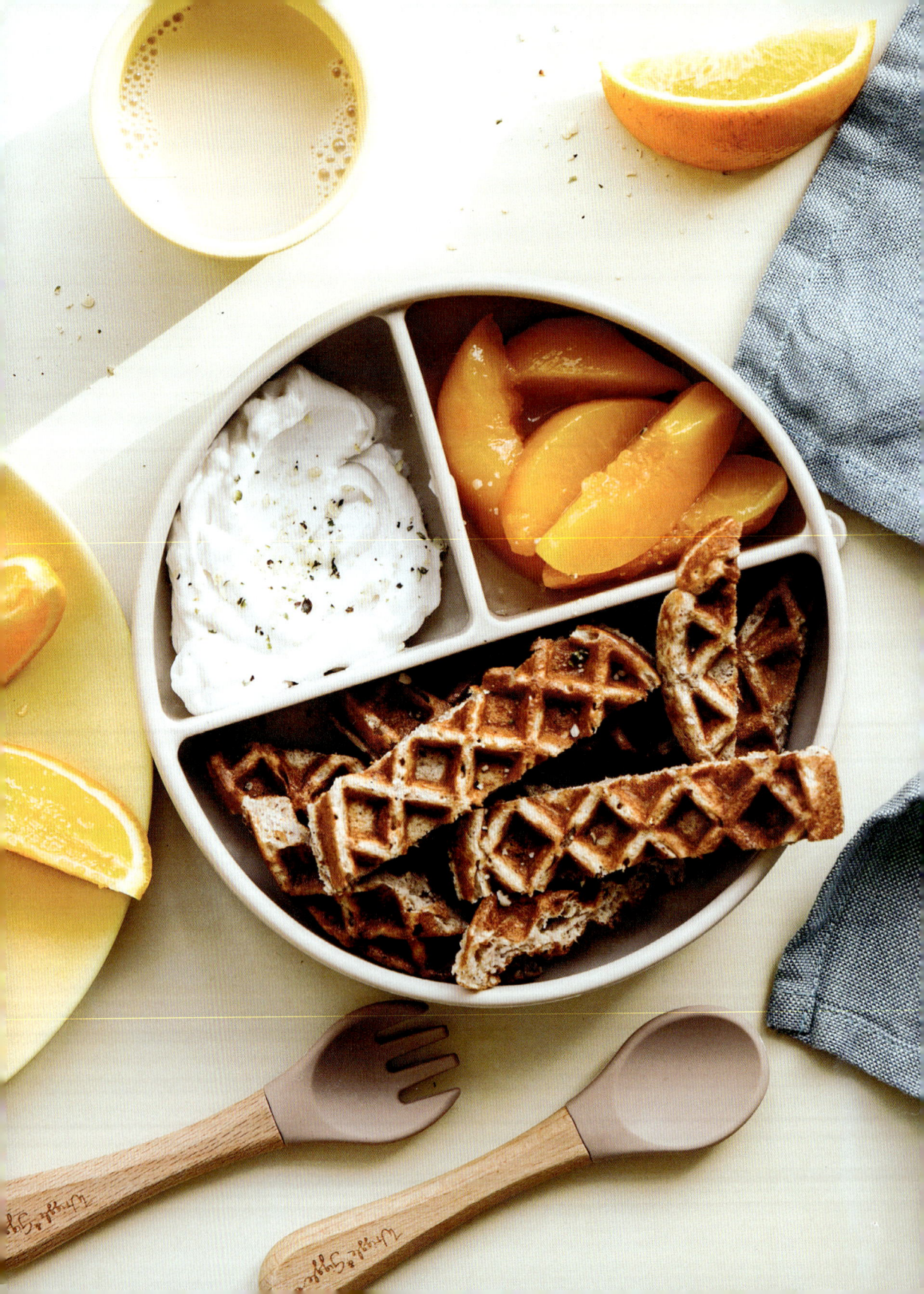

Whole-Wheat Protein Blender Waffles

My kids are always pleased to see me cooking up a batch of these deliciously crispy Whole-Wheat Protein Blender Waffles! The banana adds a natural sweetness that appeals to kids but is subtle enough that you can still drizzle over some maple syrup if desired. My top tip for getting the fluffiest, crispiest results is to not overfill your waffle iron with the batter. The waffles plump up really well, so if you add too much batter, they'll need longer to cook and may become rubbery. Less is more for this recipe!

Serves: 6

Prep Time: 5 minutes + 10 minutes to rest

Cook Time: 3 to 4 minutes per batch

INGREDIENTS

1 cup (120 g) whole-wheat flour

1 cup (90 g) rolled oats

¼ cup (25 g) ground flaxseeds

1 tsp baking powder

½ tsp baking soda

1 tsp ground cinnamon

1½ cups (420 g) plain full-fat Greek yogurt (see notes)

½ cup (120 ml) full-fat milk or milk of choice (see notes)

2 large eggs

1 large ripe banana

Nonstick cooking spray, as needed

METHOD

Add the whole-what flour, rolled oats, ground flaxseeds, baking powder, baking soda, cinnamon, Greek yogurt, milk, eggs and banana into a blender and blend on high speed for 30 seconds. Remove the blender's lid, scrape down the sides and blend again until the batter is well blended—a grainy texture is okay. Allow the batter to rest for 10 minutes—do not skip this step, as this is what makes the waffles crispy.

Preheat a waffle maker and spray it with the nonstick cooking spray. Pour in the amount of batter recommended by the waffle maker's manufacturer—erring on the side of caution to be sure not to overfill.

Cook the waffles for 3 to 4 minutes, or follow the manufacturer's instructions for your particular waffle maker, until they are golden and crispy. Remove the waffles from the waffle maker, set them aside and repeat this process with the remaining batter.

STORAGE & REHEATING

Store the waffles in an airtight container in the refrigerator for up to 3 days. To freeze them, stack the waffles between sheets of parchment paper in a freezer bag and freeze them for up to 3 months. Reheat frozen waffles in the toaster on the lowest setting until they are warmed through and crispy.

NOTES

The Greek yogurt is what adds the bulk of the protein here, so I don't recommend substituting it. However, if your child is dairy free, you can substitute it for another plain thick yogurt of your choosing, but just be aware that this will reduce the protein content of the waffles.

Feel free to use whichever milk your family prefers with the exception of oat milk, which will thicken the batter too much as it rests.

MAKE-AHEAD

FREEZER FRIENDLY

LUNCHBOX FRIENDLY

VEGETARIAN

ALLERGEN: EGG

SOURCE OF FIBER, IRON, & PROTEIN

Serves:
14

Prep Time:
7 minutes

Cook Time:
30 to 40 minutes

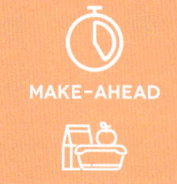

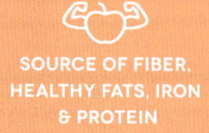

MAKE-AHEAD

LUNCHBOX FRIENDLY

VEGAN

SOURCE OF FIBER, HEALTHY FATS, IRON & PROTEIN

Toddler-Friendly Nut-Free Granola

Granola is something I always like to have on hand to sprinkle over yogurt for a super quick and nutritious breakfast or snack. It's also great for adding texture to smoothie bowls or just packing in a lunchbox to boost iron and protein. Frustratingly, most store-bought options contain high amounts of sugar, and while that's fine on occasion, I wanted to create a version that's toddler friendly, allergy friendly and contains no added sugar so it can be offered regularly. Naturally sweetened with applesauce, this recipe is super easy to pull together and makes a huge batch. You can pretty much use any seeds you prefer, and if you wish, you can add in some dried fruit and even some nuts too—the delicate coconut flavor pairs well with most dried fruits, nuts and seeds.

INGREDIENTS

2 cups (180 g) jumbo or regular sized rolled oats

½ cup (65 g) sunflower seed kernels, chopped

½ cup (50 g) unsweetened shredded or desiccated coconut

3 tbsp (30 g) hulled hemp hearts

1 tsp cinnamon

¼ tsp salt

⅓ cup (85 ml) unsweetened applesauce (if you live in the U.K., see the note on page 42)

⅓ cup (80 ml) melted coconut oil

1 tsp pure vanilla extract

ADD-INS

½ cup (75 g) roughly chopped raisins or chopped dried fruit of choice (optional)

METHOD

Preheat the oven to 350°F (180°C, gas mark 4, fan 160°C) and line a large baking sheet with parchment paper.

In a large bowl, add the rolled oats, chopped sunflower seed kernels, shredded coconut, hulled hemp hearts, cinnamon and salt and mix until well combined.

Next, add the applesauce, melted coconut oil, vanilla extract and raisins (if using) to the bowl of dry ingredients and mix until well combined, making sure all of the oat flakes and seeds are coated.

Transfer the mixture to the lined baking sheet and spread it out evenly, pressing it down with the back of a spoon as you go to create one even layer.

Bake it in the oven for 10 minutes, then stir the granola thoroughly. Flatten it again with your spoon and return it to the oven to cook for 10 more minutes. Stir the granola again, but this time do not flatten it. Cook for 10 minutes, or until lightly golden and crisp. If you want your granola to be extra golden and crispy, you can stir it again and cook it for a further 10 minutes—keep an eye on it so that it doesn't burn.

Once cooked, allow the granola to cool completely. Stir and transfer it to an airtight container. For younger toddlers who have yet to cut their molars, I recommend pulverizing their portion in a food processor before serving, as the small crunchy clusters may irritate their gums. Once your toddler has some molars, you can serve the granola as is.

STORAGE

Store in an airtight container in the refrigerator for up to 4 weeks.

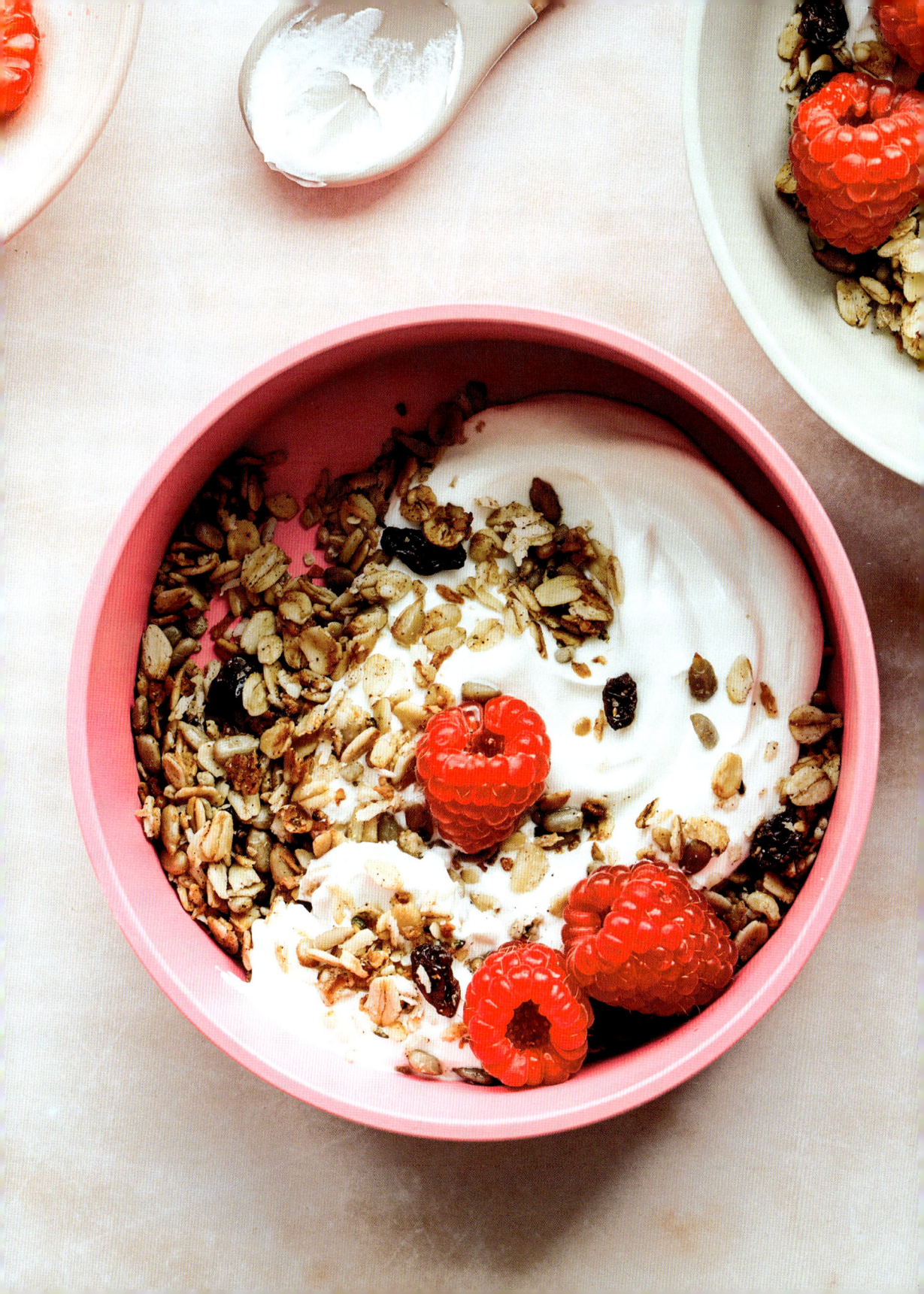

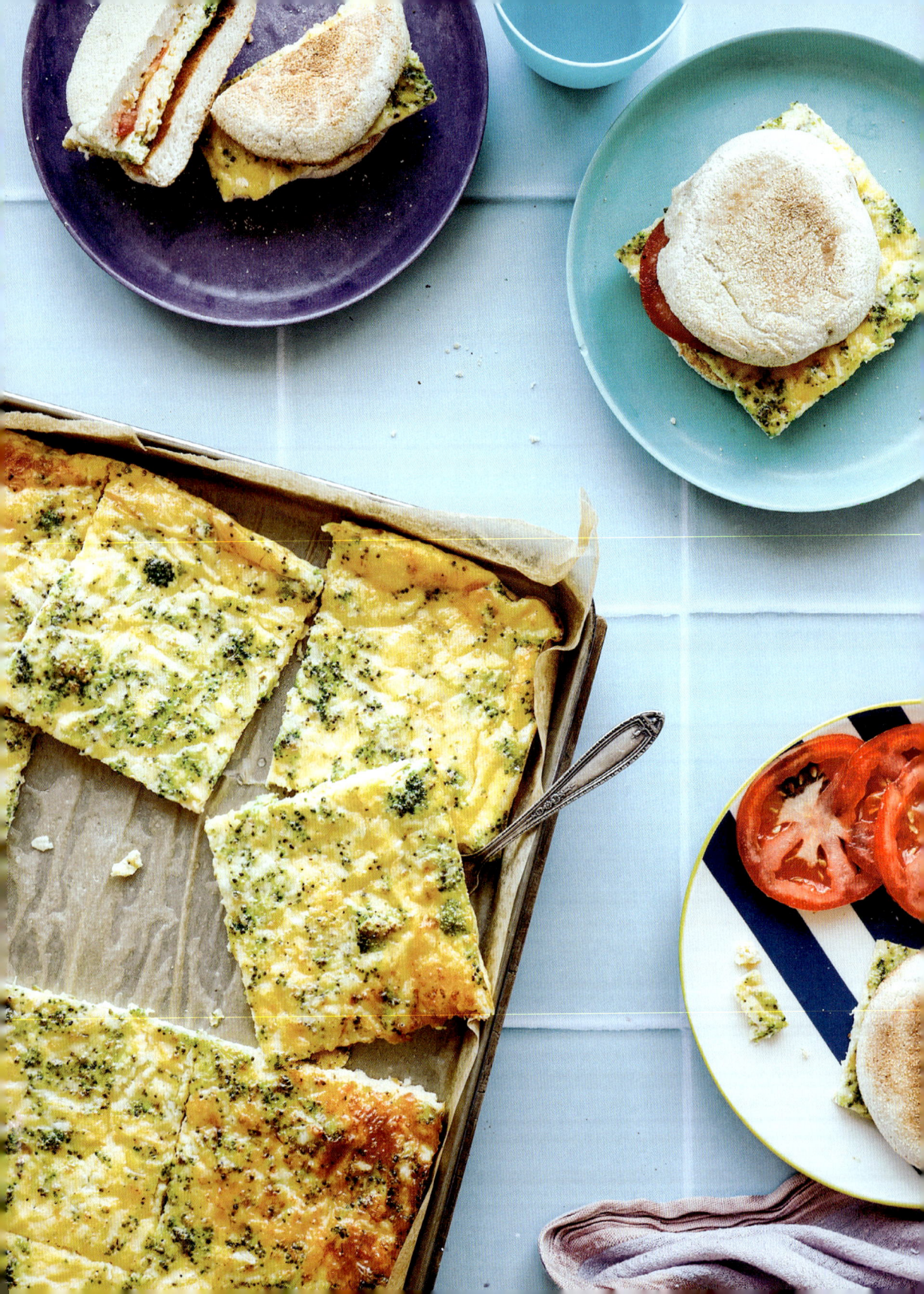

Broccoli & Cheese Sheet Pan Eggs

The humble egg! Such a versatile and nutritious food that is not only widely available, but also a more affordable iron and protein option than meat. This recipe gives you the ease of baking a frittata but with the smoother texture and flavor payoff of an omelette, and it's great for feeding a large crowd—not to mention it freezes brilliantly! This is my kids' preferred flavor combination, but you can switch up the veggies depending on what you like or what you have on hand. Just be sure to use the same ratios listed in the recipe. Our favorite way to eat them is sandwiched between a toasted buttered English muffin, often with some sliced sausage but always with a dollop of ketchup. Heavenly!

INGREDIENTS

Nonstick cooking spray, as needed

12 large eggs

½ cup (120 ml) full-fat cow's milk or nondairy milk of choice

Salt and black pepper, to taste

½ head (185 g) broccoli

1½ cups (170 g) grated cheddar cheese or nondairy cheese of choice

METHOD

Preheat the oven to 350°F (180°C, gas mark 4, fan 160°C). Line a 13 x 18-inch (33 x 45-cm) sheet pan with parchment paper and generously spray (including the sides) with the nonstick cooking spray.

In a large bowl, beat together the eggs, milk, salt and black pepper. Set aside.

Using heavy-duty kitchen scissors or a knife, proceed to "shave" the broccoli florets by snipping or cutting off the darker green part of the broccoli head, leaving the stalks behind. Add the broccoli shavings to the egg mixture and mix to combine.

Pour the mixture into the prepared sheet pan and sprinkle the cheddar cheese over the top. Carefully place the sheet pan on the middle shelf in the oven. Cook for 18 to 20 minutes, or until the eggs are fully set. Allow to cool slightly before cutting the egg sheet into twelve squares.

STORAGE

Store the sliced egg squares in an airtight container in the refrigerator for up to 3 days. To freeze, stack the cooled egg squares between sheets of parchment paper in a freezer bag and freeze them for up to 3 months.

Serves: **12**

Prep Time: **8 minutes**

Cook Time: **18 to 20 minutes**

30 — READY IN 30 MINUTES OR LESS

MAKE-AHEAD

FREEZER FRIENDLY

VEGETARIAN

ALLERGEN: EGG

SOURCE OF IRON & PROTEIN

Serves:
4

Prep Time:
6 minutes

Cook Time:
3 to 6 minutes per batch

READY IN 30 MINUTES OR LESS

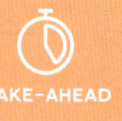

MAKE-AHEAD

FREEZER FRIENDLY

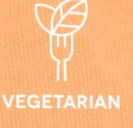

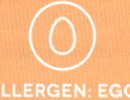

VEGETARIAN

ALLERGEN: EGG

Fluffy Applesauce Pancakes

These pillowy soft, light and fluffy applesauce pancakes are the perfect weekend breakfast, and the batter comes together in one bowl in mere minutes! You can use either store-bought or homemade applesauce here—both will do a wonderful job of adding subtle apple flavor while naturally sweetening the pancakes, making them perfect to eat plain or with maple syrup. If you want to change up the flavor, you can replace the vanilla extract with ½ teaspoon of ground cinnamon, which is the perfect combination for those crisp fall mornings.

INGREDIENTS

¾ cup (95 g) all-purpose flour

1 tsp baking powder

½ cup (130 g) unsweetened applesauce (see notes)

1 large egg

¼ cup (60 ml) full-fat milk or nondairy milk of choice

2 tbsp (30 ml) melted butter or coconut oil

1 tsp pure vanilla extract

Nonstick cooking spray, as needed

METHOD

In a large bowl, combine the flour and baking powder. Make a well in the center of the dry ingredients and add the applesauce, egg, milk, melted butter and vanilla extract. Using a wooden spoon, gently beat the ingredients together until you have a smooth batter, being careful not to overmix.

Heat a large nonstick frying pan over medium heat. Spray the frying pan with the nonstick cooking spray. Add ¼-cup (60-ml) dollops of the batter to the frying pan. Cook the pancakes for 2 to 4 minutes, until bubbles form across the pancakes and the undersides are golden. Flip the pancakes and cook them for 1 to 2 minutes, or until the bottoms are golden. Remove the pancakes from the frying pan, set them aside and repeat this process with the remaining batter.

STORAGE & REHEATING

Store the pancakes in an airtight container in the refrigerator for up to 3 days. To freeze them, stack the pancakes between sheets of parchment paper in a freezer bag and freeze them for up to 3 months.

Reheat frozen pancakes by placing them in an even layer on a large baking sheet. Cover them with a baking sheet or aluminium foil and heat them in the oven at 350°F (180°C, gas mark 4, fan 160°C) for 10 minutes, until they are warm and soft.

NOTES

If you are in the United Kingdom, please note that the applesauce referenced in this recipe is pureed apples, not the chunky applesauce you typically find in the condiment section at the supermarket. Applesauce is now widely available in the U.K., but if you're having trouble finding it, be sure to check out the baby aisle for the apple puree pouches, which are the same thing, just in smaller quantities.

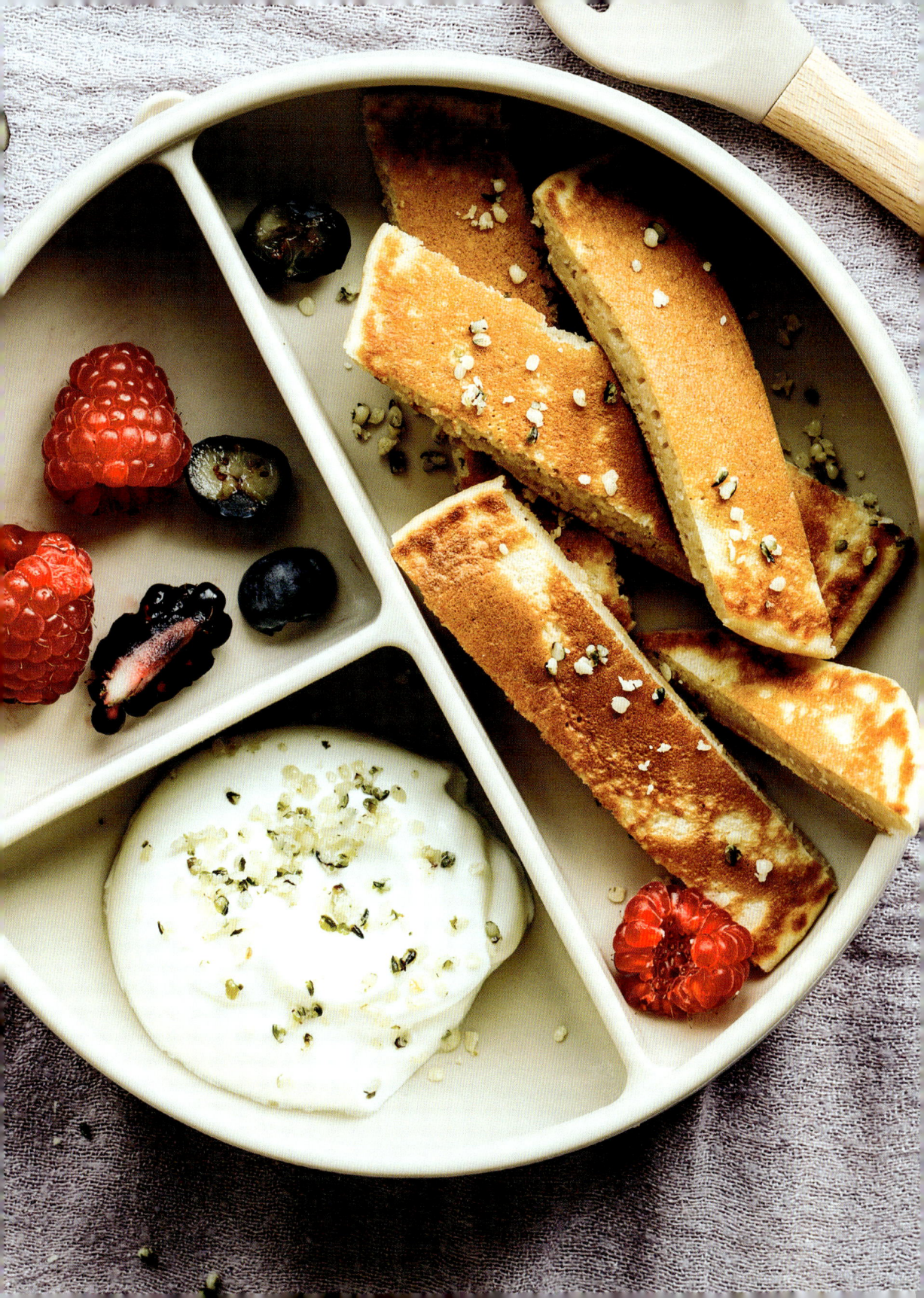

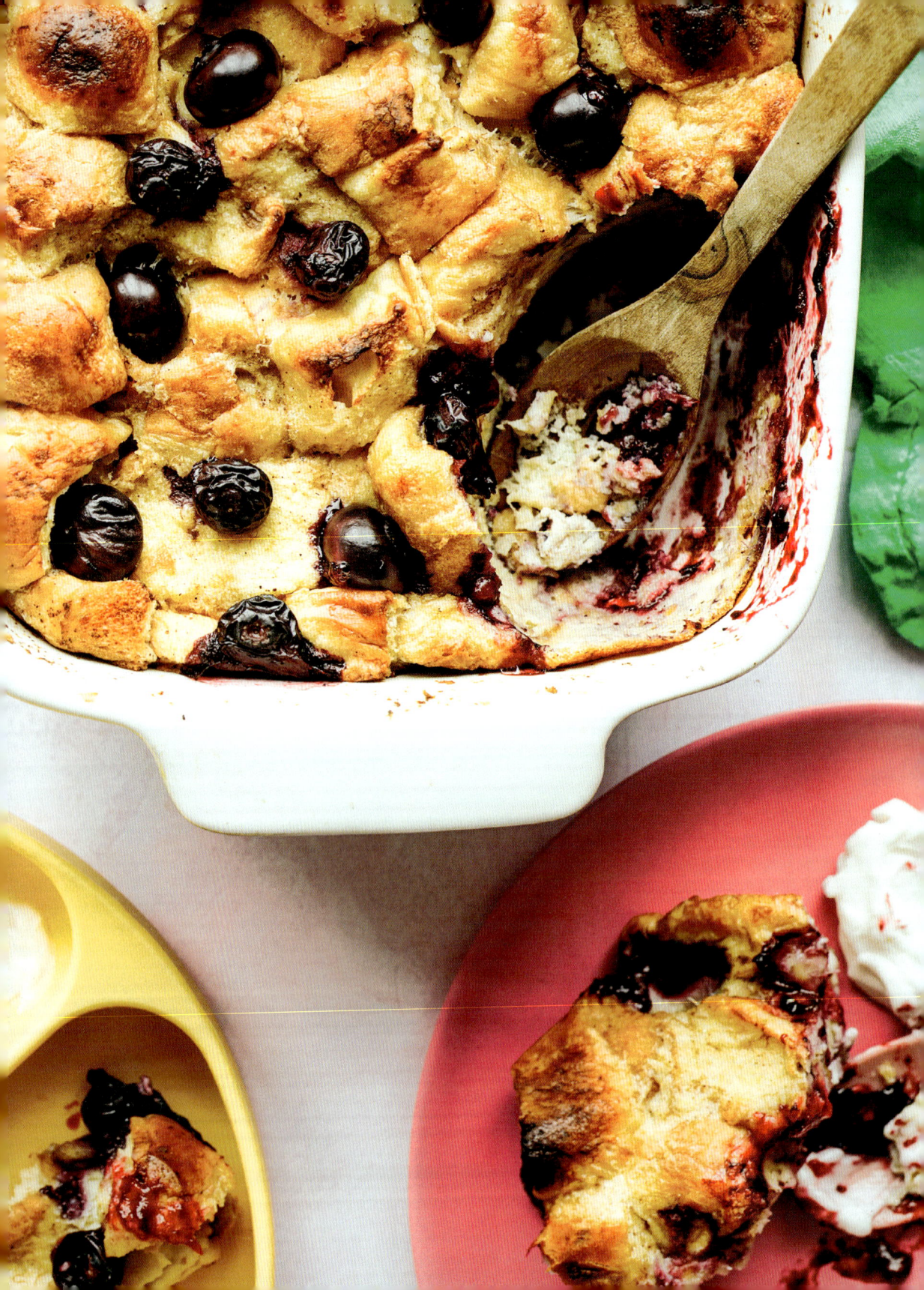

Blueberry & Banana French Toast Bake

I am in love with this recipe! For me, it's the perfect cross between French toast and bread and butter pudding, and the pillowy, yet crispy texture feels like such a decadent weekend treat. My younger kids are convinced we are eating dessert for breakfast!

My favorite thing about this recipe is that it can be made the night before, so when I wake up, all I have to do is pop it into the oven and breakfast is served—this really speaks to my busy mom heart because life has been so chaotic lately. Feel free to switch out the blueberries for another berry of choice, or you could even add some dried chopped fruit—raisins work very well here. The rich and buttery brioche is what gives this recipe its decadent feel. It soaks up the custard beautifully, but you can use another bread if desired. I recommend thickly sliced sourdough bread or French bread as alternatives, just be aware that using different breads will change the texture.

Serves: 8

Prep Time: 10 minutes + 30 minutes to soak

Cook Time: 40 to 45 minutes

INGREDIENTS

- 2 small ripe bananas, or 1 large banana
- 2 cups (480 ml) full-fat cow's milk or nondairy milk of choice
- 4 large eggs
- 1 tsp pure vanilla extract
- ½ tsp cinnamon
- ¼ tsp salt
- 1 (14-oz [400-g]) loaf brioche bread, cut into 1-inch (2.5-cm) cubes or bread of choice (see recipe introduction for suggestions)
- ½ cup (75 g) fresh or frozen blueberries

METHOD

Add the bananas to a medium-sized baking dish and mash well with a fork. Add the milk, eggs, vanilla extract, cinnamon and salt and whisk together until well combined.

Add the cubed brioche bread to the custard mixture and gently stir the bread until all the bread cubes are coated and beginning to soak up the custard. Cover and refrigerate for at least 30 minutes or preferably overnight.

Preheat the oven to 375°F (190°C, gas mark 5, fan 170°C) 10 minutes before you are ready to bake the soaked brioche bread. Remove the baking dish from the refrigerator and scatter the blueberries evenly over the top.

Cover the baking dish with a baking sheet or aluminium foil and bake in the oven for 30 minutes. Uncover and bake for 10 to 15 minutes more, or until the top is golden brown and crispy and the French toast is set.

STORAGE & REHEATING

Store in an airtight container in the refrigerator for up to 3 days. To reheat, place the leftover French toast bake (covered with a baking sheet or aluminium foil) in the oven at 350°F (180°C, gas mark 4, fan 160°C) for 20 to 25 minutes, or until warmed through. Alternatively, you can reheat individual servings in the microwave on the high setting for 30-second intervals until warmed through.

MAKE-AHEAD

FREEZER FRIENDLY

VEGETARIAN

ALLERGEN: EGG

SOURCE OF IRON & PROTEIN

Serves:
2

Prep Time:
5 minutes

Easy Peachy Smoothie Bowl

My kids are obsessed with smoothie bowls, and I love how simple yet delicious this recipe is; no frills and nothing fancy, just simple and nutritious ingredients that transform into a beautifully silky smoothie bowl that carry the delicate sweet and floral flavors of peach with ease. You may be tempted to skip the orange juice here, but I urge you not to, as the sharp citrusy flavor helps to balance out the mellow notes of the peach and gives the smoothie a subtle but welcoming kick. Although the yogurt provides a good amount of fat to keep little tummies full, I often double down and serve this smoothie bowl with a generous sprinkling of my Toddler-Friendly Nut-Free Granola (page 38), which also adds great texture and crunch!

INGREDIENTS

2 cups (240 g) frozen peeled peach or nectarine slices

1 frozen medium ripe banana

½ cup (140 g) full-fat plain Greek yogurt or plain coconut yogurt

⅓ cup (80 ml) orange juice, plus more as needed

METHOD

Add all of the ingredients into a blender and blend on high speed for 30 seconds. Remove the blender's lid, scrape down the sides and blend again until smooth, adding more orange juice to loosen up the smoothie as needed. If you'd like to make this smoothie into a drink, keep adding liquid (orange juice or water) until you reach your desired consistency.

STORAGE

Leftovers can be frozen into popsicle molds for a quick and refreshing snack.

READY IN 30 MINUTES OR LESS

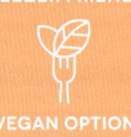

FREEZER FRIENDLY

VEGAN OPTION

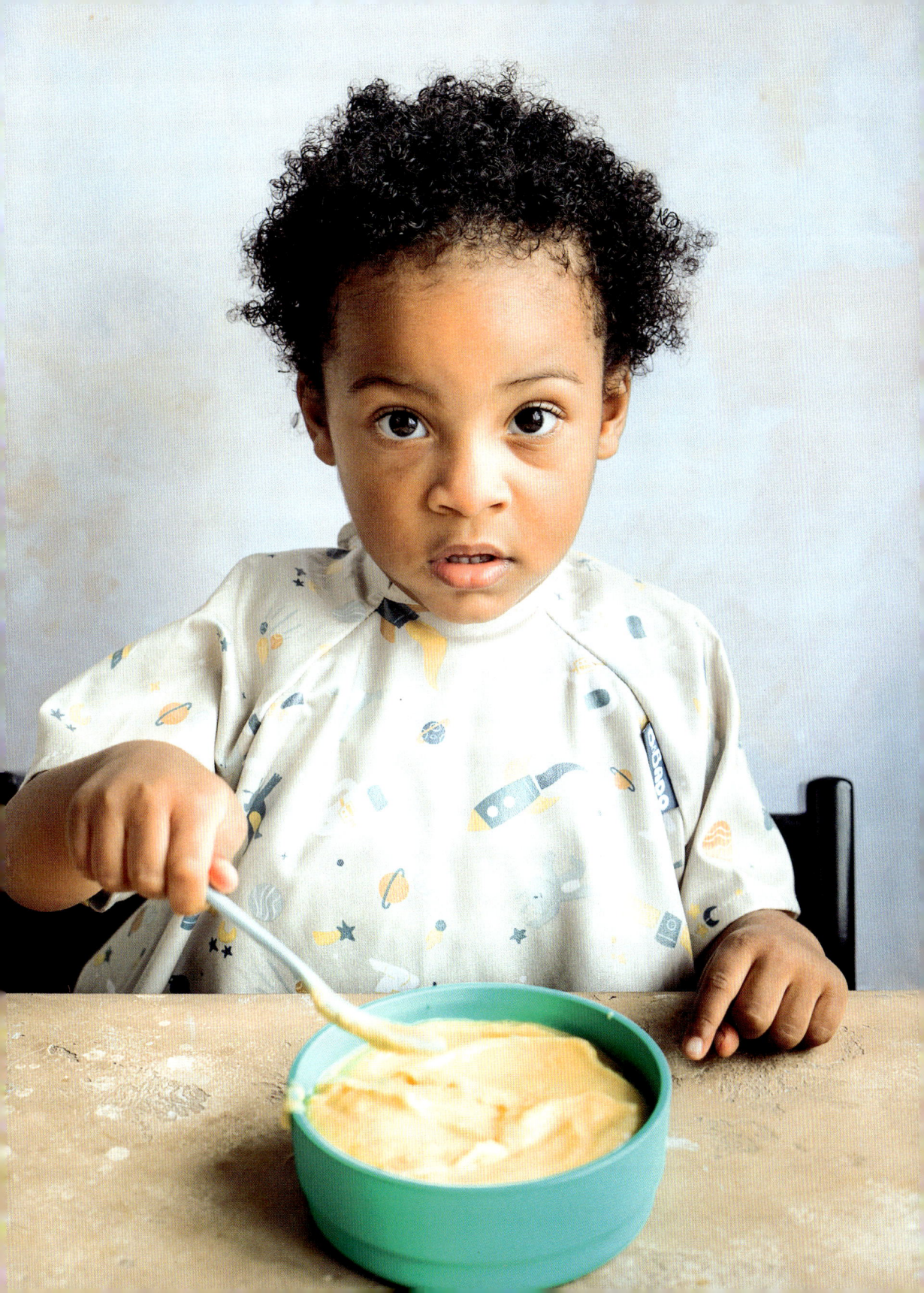

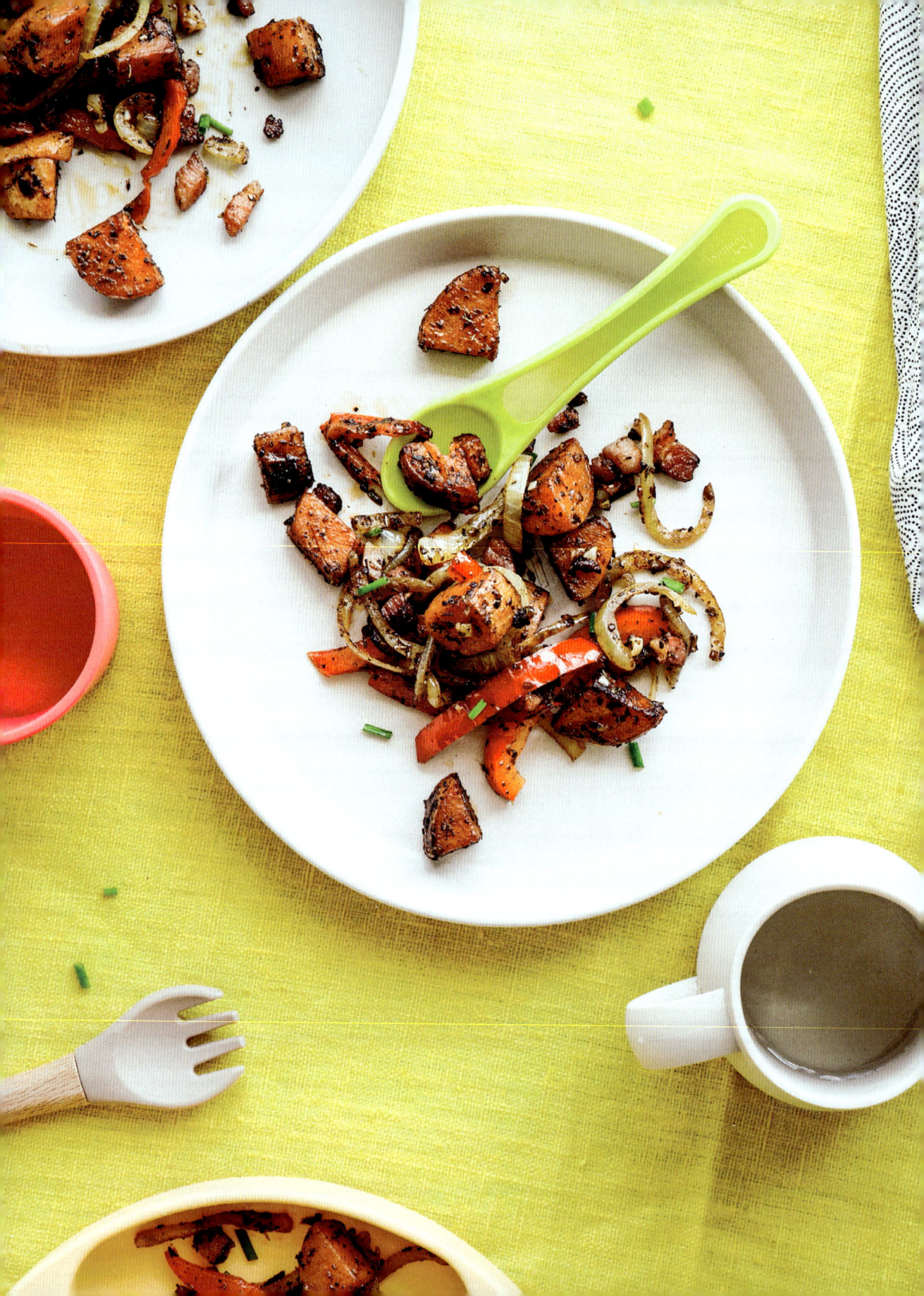

Sweet Potato Breakfast Hash

Make way for this delicious weekend delight, which is perfect for breakfast or lunch, or even as a side dish for dinner. This sweet potato breakfast hash is absolutely bursting with flavor and will appeal to the whole family. The onion, red pepper and garlic merge perfectly with the sweet, salty, smokiness of the bacon, and frying the naturally sweet potatoes in the bacon fat gives them an incredible depth of flavor, which is further complemented by the smoked paprika and herby oregano. I recommend serving this with fried or scrambled eggs for a hearty and filling meal.

Serves: 4

Prep Time: 10 minutes

Cook Time: 30 to 35 minutes

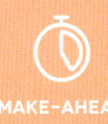

INGREDIENTS

2 tbsp (30 ml) avocado or olive oil, plus more as needed

1 small brown onion, halved and thinly sliced

1 small red bell pepper, deseeded and finely diced

3.5 oz (100 g) bacon lardons or pancetta

2 garlic cloves, minced

2 large sweet potatoes, peeled and cut into ½-inch (1-cm) cubes

½ tsp smoked paprika

1 tsp oregano

Salt and black pepper, to taste

2 tbsp (6 g) chopped fresh chives (optional)

METHOD

Heat a large nonstick frying pan over medium-high heat and add 2 tablespoons (30 ml) of the avocado oil. Once the oil is hot, add the sliced onion and diced red bell pepper and sauté for 2 to 3 minutes, until they start to soften.

Add the bacon lardons and cook for 2 to 3 minutes, stirring often. Once the bacon starts to crisp up, add the minced garlic and cook for 1 minute. Use a slotted spoon to remove everything from the pan (leaving the cooking fat behind) and set aside.

If needed, add some more avocado oil to the pan, then add the diced sweet potatoes, smoked paprika, oregano, salt and black pepper and mix until everything is well combined and the potatoes are coated in the oil. Cover, turn the heat down to medium and cook for 10 minutes, stirring halfway through. Remove the lid and cook for 2 to 3 minutes, or until the potatoes start to become golden and crispy.

Add the bacon and vegetable mix back to the pan and mix to combine. Cook for 2 to 3 minutes to let all the flavors infuse and let the sweet potatoes finish cooking, stirring and tossing often. Garnish with chopped chives (if using) before serving.

STORAGE & REHEATING

Store leftovers in an airtight container in the refrigerator for up to 3 days. To reheat, place the sweet potato hash in a baking dish and reheat (covered) at 350°F (180°C, gas mark 4, fan 160°C) for 10 to 15 minutes, or until heated through. Alternatively, you can reheat individual servings in the microwave (covered) on the high setting for 30-second intervals until warmed through.

MAKE-AHEAD

SOURCE OF IRON & PROTEIN

Serves: 4

Prep Time: 5 minutes

Cook Time: 18 to 22 minutes

- READY IN 30 MINUTES OR LESS
- MAKE-AHEAD
- FREEZER FRIENDLY
- LUNCHBOX FRIENDLY
- VEGETARIAN
- ALLERGEN: EGG
- SOURCE OF FIBER, IRON & PROTEIN

Breakfast Banana Cake Cups

Bananas and oats feature in a lot of my baking and breakfast ideas, and I often wonder if I am sharing too many recipes with similar ingredients, but then I remember that the reality of life is that we often have the same ingredients on hand. Often, its more useful to learn how to use these ingredients in different ways than it is to stress ourselves out by trying to create fancy new meals with a ton of different ingredients every day. These Breakfast Banana Cake Cups are iron and protein rich and a quicker alternative to regular banana bread that comes together in the blender with such ease.

The individual portions mean that you can get creative with the toppings, making sure there is something for everyone. I often make these in advance and freeze them, as they can be thawed in the microwave in less than a minute. They're such a great mess-free way to eat oats in the morning, and I usually serve them with a glass of milk and some extra fruit on the side.

INGREDIENTS

Nonstick cooking spray, as needed

1 cup (90 g) rolled oats

1 tsp baking powder

½ tsp cinnamon

2 large eggs

2 small overripe bananas, or 1 large overripe banana

1 tsp pure vanilla extract

¼ cup (45 g) chocolate chips, raisins or chopped berries of choice, for topping

METHOD

Preheat the oven to 350°F (180°C, gas mark 4, fan 160°C) and spray four small ramekins with the nonstick cooking spray.

Add the rolled oats, baking powder, cinnamon, eggs, bananas and vanilla extract to a blender or food processor and blend on high speed for 30 seconds. Remove the blender lid, scrape down the sides and blend again until the batter is well blended. Divide the mixture evenly between the ramekins and distribute your toppings of choice on top.

Bake in the oven for 18 to 22 minutes, or until they are golden brown and a toothpick inserted into the center of a cake cup comes out clean of wet batter. Allow to cool slightly before serving.

STORAGE & REHEATING

Store the cakes in an airtight container in the refrigerator for up to 3 days. To freeze, place the cooled cakes in a freezer bag in an even layer and freeze them for up to 3 months. Thaw the cakes in the refrigerator, at room temperature or in the microwave on the high setting for 30 to 60 seconds. Frozen cakes can be packed in a lunchbox, and they will thaw in 1 to 2 hours.

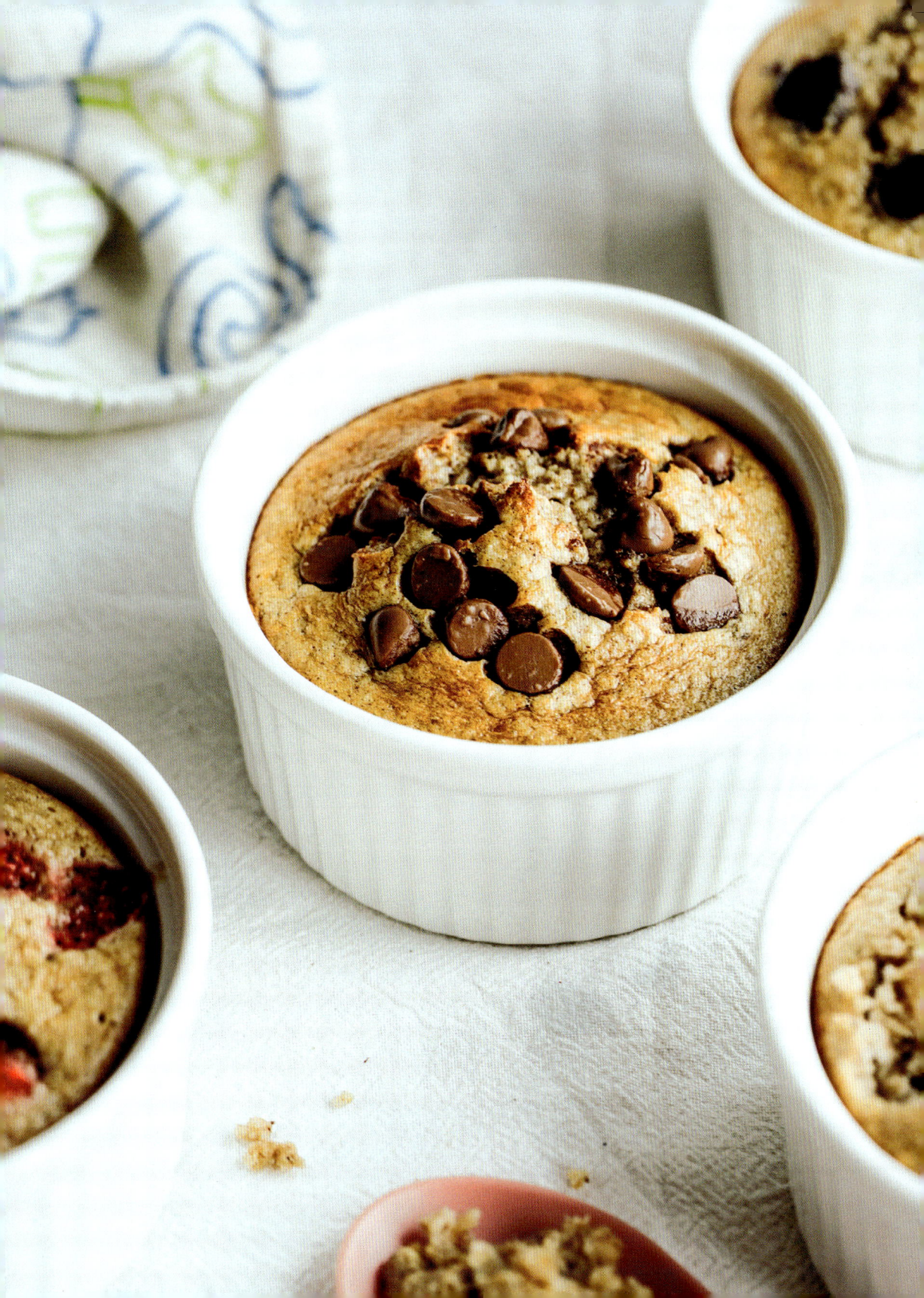

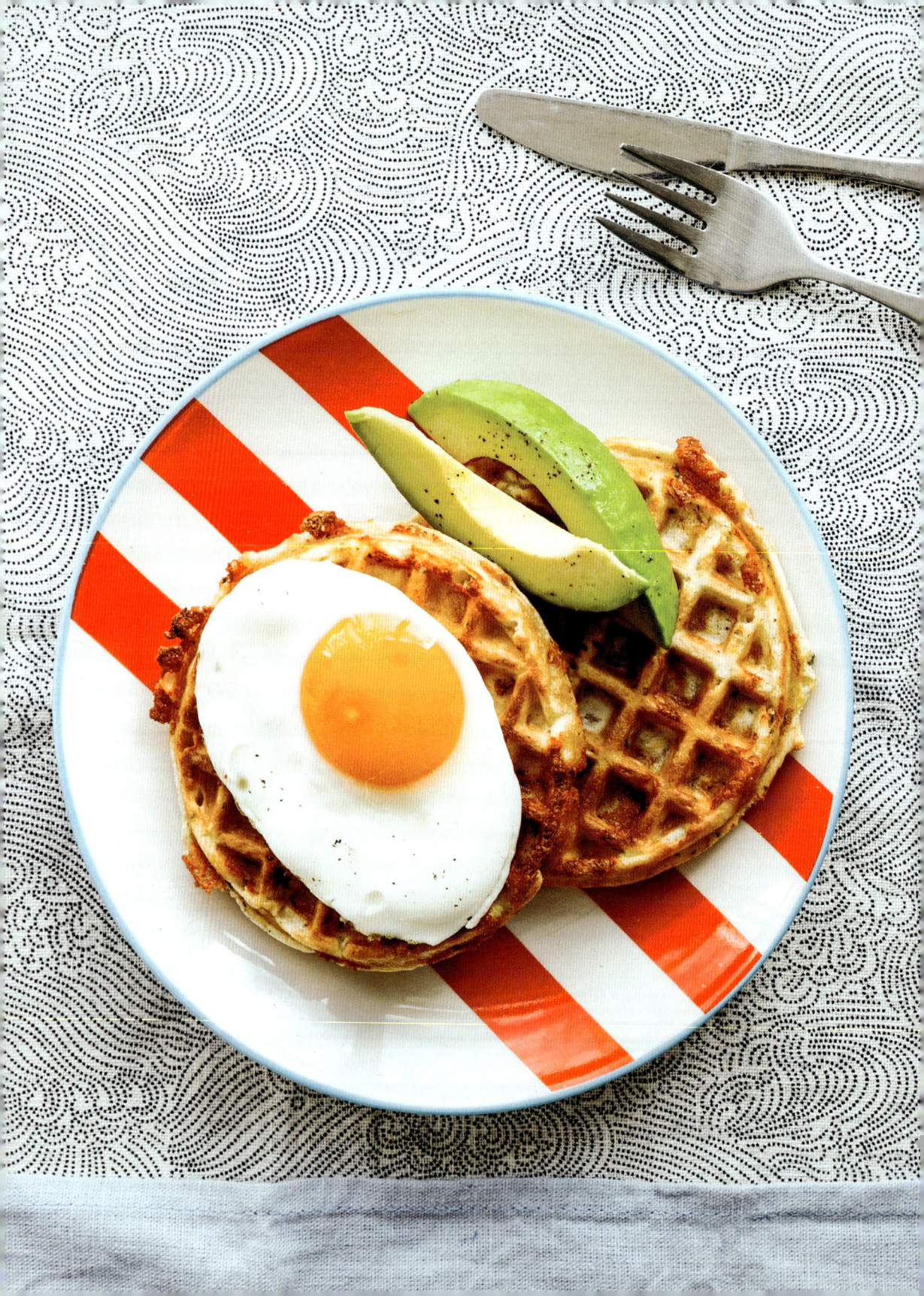

Savory Cheddar Waffles

A waffle can be pretty much anything you want it to be, and this savory cheesy version is a must-have in your breakfast or lunch rotation. The sharp cheddar creates a crispy cheesiness that is so moreish and is the perfect companion to eggs. You can also ramp up the flavors by adding some finely chopped spring onion or crispy cooked bacon to the batter mix—I often add both of these to half the batter mix for some variety. They also freeze really well and can be heated from frozen in the toaster for super quick and easy breakfasts or lunches on those busy days!

INGREDIENTS

- 2 large eggs
- ¾ cup (180 ml) full-fat cow's milk or milk of choice
- ½ cup (140 g) full-fat plain Greek yogurt
- 2 tbsp (30 ml) melted unsalted butter
- 1 tsp onion granules or onion powder
- 2 tsp (2 g) dried mixed herbs
- 1½ cups (190 g) all-purpose flour
- 1 tsp baking powder
- 1½ cups (170 g) grated cheddar cheese

METHOD

In a large bowl, add the eggs, milk, Greek yogurt, melted butter, onion granules and mixed herbs. Whisk together until well combined.

Add the flour and baking powder and using a wooden spoon, mix until well combined, being careful not to overmix—a few lumps are okay. Fold in the grated cheese.

Preheat a waffle maker and spray it with the nonstick cooking spray. Pour in the amount of batter recommended by the waffle maker's manufacturer.

Cook the waffles for 3 to 4 minutes, until they are golden and crispy, or follow the manufacturer's instructions for your particular waffle maker. Remove the waffles from the waffle maker, set them aside and repeat this process with the remaining batter.

STOAGE & REHEATING

Store the waffles in an airtight container in the refrigerator for up to 3 days. To freeze them, stack the waffles between sheets of parchment paper in a freezer bag and freeze them for up to 3 months. Reheat frozen waffles in the toaster on the lowest setting until they are warmed through and crispy.

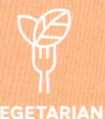

Serves: 6

Prep Time: 8 minutes

Cook Time: 3 to 4 minutes per batch

- MAKE-AHEAD
- FREEZER FRIENDLY
- LUNCHBOX FRIENDLY
- VEGETARIAN
- ALLERGEN: DAIRY & EGG
- SOURCE OF IRON & PROTEIN

Serves:
2

Prep Time:
5 minutes

Cook Time:
10 minutes

READY IN 30 MINUTES OR LESS

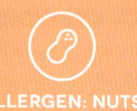

VEGAN

ALLERGEN: NUTS

SOURCE OF FIBER, HEALTHY FATS, IRON & PROTEIN

Iron-Rich Banana & Cashew Oatmeal

I am so excited to share this oatmeal recipe because it's been on heavy rotation in my home for well over a year! I created this combination when I was weaning my youngest son onto solids, as I wanted to maximize his iron intake, which is a critical nutrient for both babies and toddlers. Besides the banana, every ingredient used in this recipe is a fantastic iron source! Cashew butter is smoother and creamier than other nut butters, which makes this oatmeal so deliciously decadent, but if you can't find it, you can use almond or peanut butter instead.

Similarly with cashew milk, you can use almond milk instead, if needed. Speaking of cashew milk, it can be on the pricey side, so I recommend freezing the leftover milk in individual portions for the next time you make this oatmeal—that way, you will not be wasting any of that creamy, nutritious and tasty milk! To serve, I like to add chopped strawberries on top—not only is this a tasty combination, but also strawberries are rich in vitamin C, which helps the body to absorb more of the iron from the oatmeal.

INGREDIENTS

1 cup (90 g) rolled oats

2 tbsp (20 g) hulled hemp hearts

1 medium ripe banana, mashed

1 cup (240 ml) cashew milk, divided, plus more as needed

2 tbsp (30 g) smooth cashew butter

METHOD

Heat a medium pan over medium-high heat and add the oats, hulled hemp hearts, mashed banana, ½ cup (120 ml) of the cashew milk and the cashew butter. Stir everything together until well combined and bring to a boil. Turn the heat down to medium-low and continuously stir for around 4 to 5 minutes as the oatmeal cooks. Add the remainder of the cashew milk bit by bit as needed as the oatmeal thickens. Feel free to use more should you need to.

Once the oatmeal has reached your desired texture and consistency, remove from the heat and allow to cool sufficiently before serving.

STORAGE

Best served fresh, but leftovers can be stored in an airtight container in the refrigerator for up to 2 days.

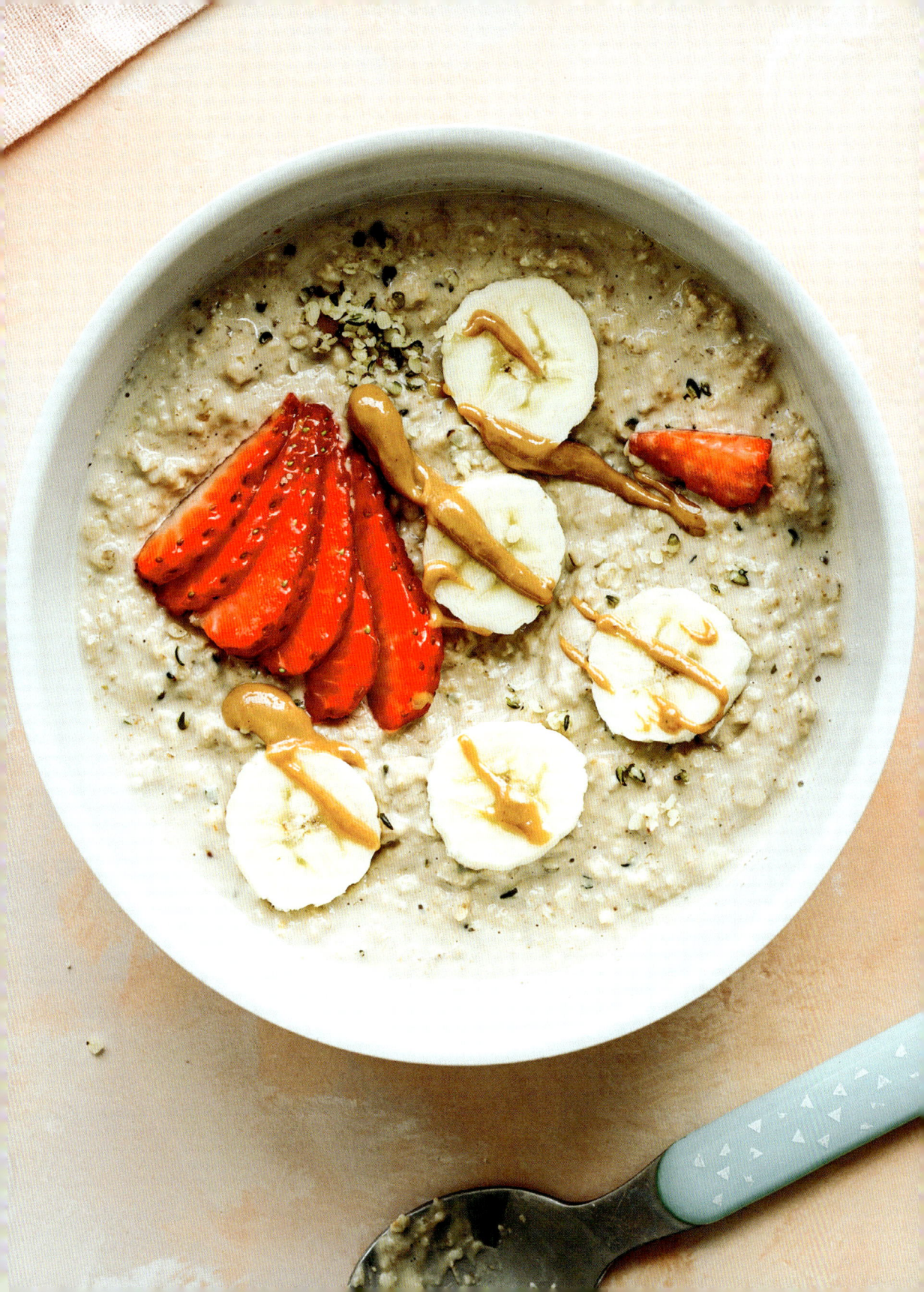

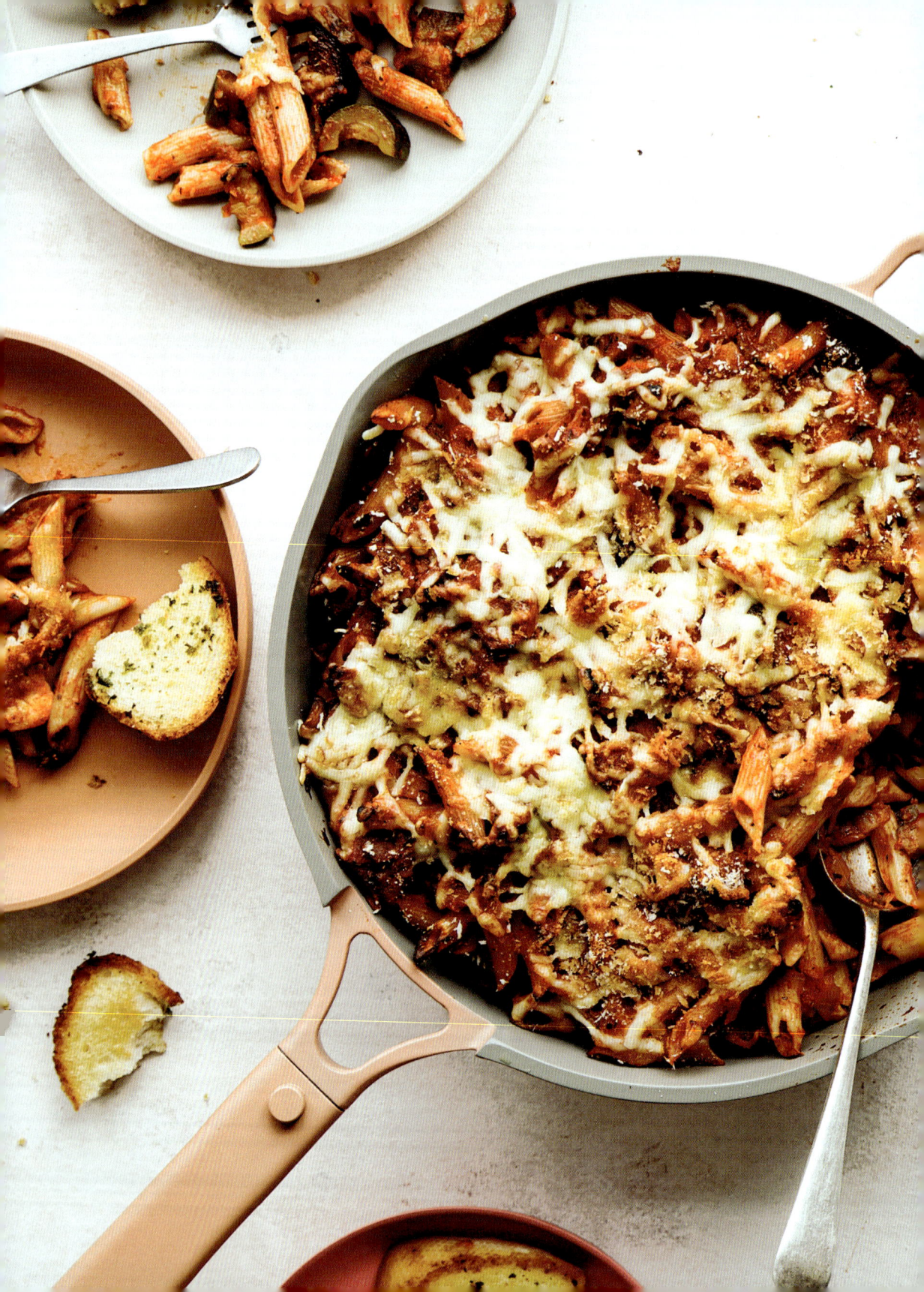

CHAPTER 4

Nutritious & Delicious Mains that Little Ones Will Love

In this chapter, you will find a selection of nutritious and tasty main meals that can be served for either lunch or dinner—all of which are either quick to prepare or simple to throw together. I have included a variety of meat, vegetarian and vegan recipes, along with many iron-rich options. Please note that for many of the recipes, the portion sizes are on the generous side to allow you to offer your toddler leftovers the next day or freeze for a later date.

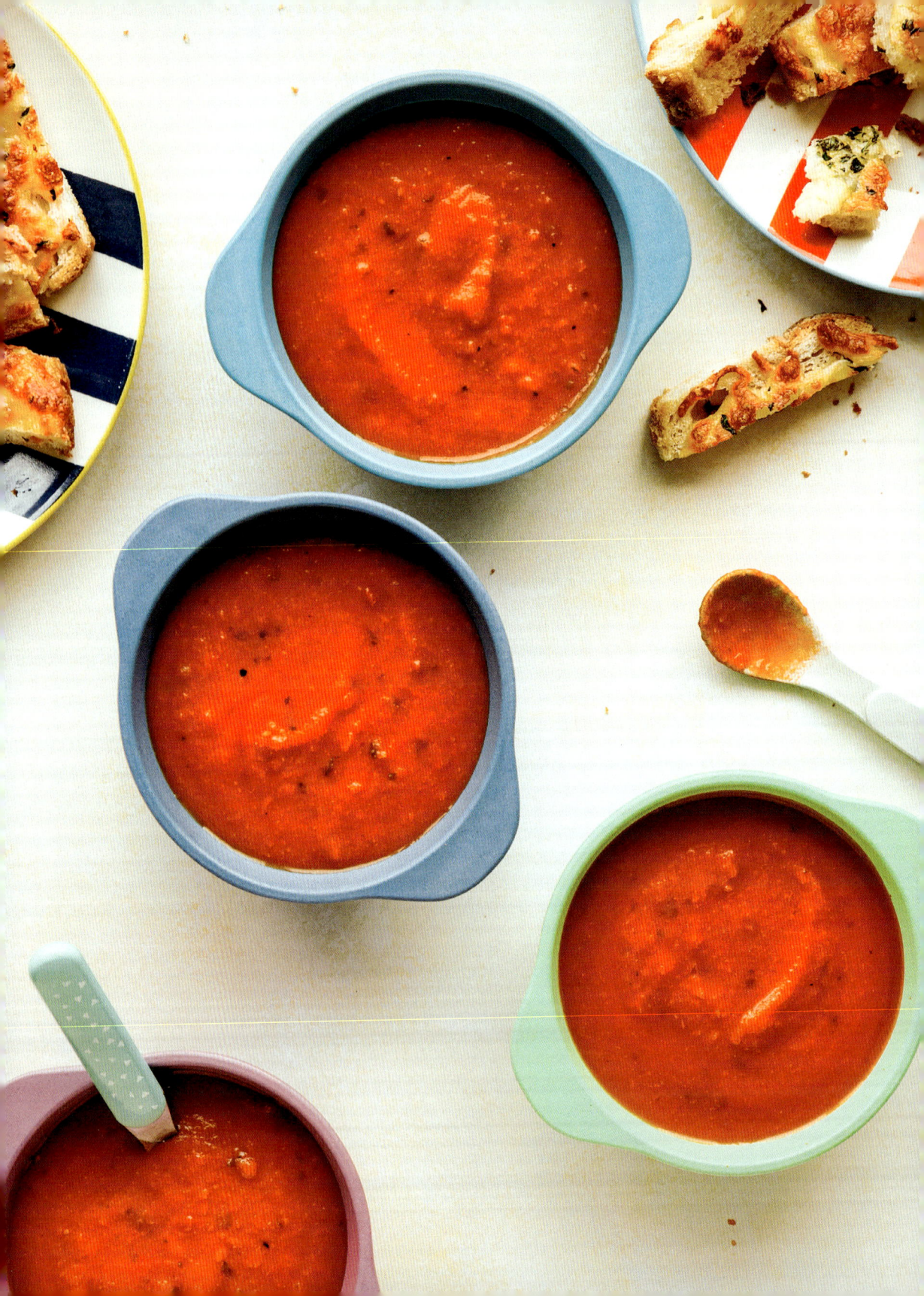

20-Minute Iron-Rich Tomato Soup

Most kids love tomato soup, and while the store-bought options are great, this super quick homemade version offers the added benefit of being lower in sugar and has an added boost of iron and protein, thanks to the white beans! What's more, the white beans effortlessly add body to the soup, meaning you get that silky, creamy texture without adding heavy cream. Perfect if your little one is dairy free! This soup pairs perfectly with my Cheesy Garlic Bread (page 108).

Serves: 4

Prep Time: 4 minutes

Cook Time: 16 minutes

INGREDIENTS

3 tbsp (45 g) butter or 2 tbsp (30 ml) olive oil

1 large red onion, finely chopped

2 garlic cloves, minced

Salt and black pepper, to taste

2 (15-oz [400-g]) cans chopped tomatoes, undrained (see notes)

¼ cup (60 g) tomato paste

1 (15 oz [400 g]) can cannellini beans, rinsed

4 cups (960 ml) vegetable broth

1 cup (25 g) lightly packed fresh basil, roughly torn

METHOD

Heat a large pot over medium-low heat and add the butter. Once the butter has melted, add the chopped onion and sauté for 4 minutes, stirring often. Add the minced garlic, salt and black pepper to the pan and cook for 1 minute.

Add the chopped tomatoes, tomato paste, cannellini beans and vegetable broth to the pan, mix to combine and bring to a boil. Turn the heat down to low, cover and simmer for 8 minutes.

Add the fresh basil to the soup and mix to combine. Put the lid back on and simmer for 2 minutes.

Turn off the heat and, using an immersion (stick) blender, blend the soup until smooth. Alternatively, you can blend the soup in a blender or food processor. To do this safely, you must blend the soup in batches, and blend on the low setting with a tea towel placed on top of the blender. Be very careful as the hot soup will expand when blending and may spit.

STORAGE & REHEATING

Store the cooled soup in an airtight container in the refrigerator for up to 3 days. To freeze, divide the soup into individual portions (if desired) and freeze for up to 3 months. Defrost the soup overnight in the refrigerator before reheating on the stove. Alternatively, you can reheat the soup from frozen on the stove with a splash of water, breaking it up with a spoon as it warms through.

NOTES

For this recipe, I recommend using the best quality canned tomatoes your budget will allow. The better quality the canned tomatoes, the better the results will be. Cheaper varieties tend to be waterier and may change the consistency or texture of the soup, as well as the acidity.

30 READY IN 30 MINUTES OR LESS

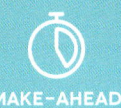

MAKE-AHEAD

FREEZER FRIENDLY

VEGAN OPTION

SOURCE OF IRON & PROTEIN

Serves:
4

Prep Time:
5 minutes + 10 minutes to marinate

Cook Time:
40 to 50 minutes

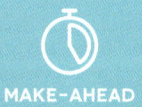

MAKE-AHEAD

FREEZER FRIENDLY

LUNCHBOX FRIENDLY

SOURCE OF IRON & PROTEIN

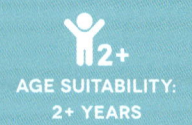

AGE SUITABILITY: 2+ YEARS

Smoky Honey Chicken Drumsticks

Chicken drumsticks are a great option for dinner. They come fully prepped and are pretty low effort when it comes to cooking them, but if done incorrectly, drumsticks can lack flavor and become incredibly dry or, even worse, dry on the inside but with slimy skin on the outside. This recipe is my foolproof way of adding maximum flavor to drumsticks while retaining the juices and creating a fabulously crispy exterior. The trick here is to leave the skin on, as this helps to retain those flavorful juices, and crisp the skin up by cooking them on a wire rack so the steam can escape.

I like to use smoked paprika to season the drumsticks, as it's a kid-friendly spice that provides deep but subtle flavor with just the tiniest bit of heat, which is generally undetectable to kids. The honey provides an additional layer of subtle sweetness and a delectable stickiness that gets even meat-hating kids interested. You can skip the honey for kids under 2 if desired, and honey must never be served to babies under 1, even when cooked.

INGREDIENTS

8 chicken drumsticks (see notes for serving tips)

2 tsp (5 g) smoked paprika

1 tsp garlic granules or powder

1 tsp onion granules or powder

Salt and black pepper, to taste

1 tbsp (15 ml) avocado or olive oil

2 tbsp (30 ml) clear runny honey

METHOD

Preheat the oven to 425°F (220°C, gas mark 7, fan 200°C) and line a large rimmed baking sheet or dish with parchment paper. Place a wire rack on top of the parchment paper.

Pat the chicken drumsticks dry with paper towels, then add them to a large bowl along with the smoked paprika, garlic granules, onion granules, salt, black pepper and avocado oil. Mix thoroughly until all the drumsticks are coated in the seasonings. Set aside to marinate for 10 minutes.

Add the honey to the chicken and mix again until all the drumsticks are evenly coated. Lay the drumsticks on a wire rack on the lined baking tray, spacing them out so that they are not overlapping.

Bake uncovered in the oven for 40 to 50 minutes, turning halfway through until the skin is slightly charred and crispy. The chicken is cooked through when the juices run clear when pierced with a fork.

(Continued)

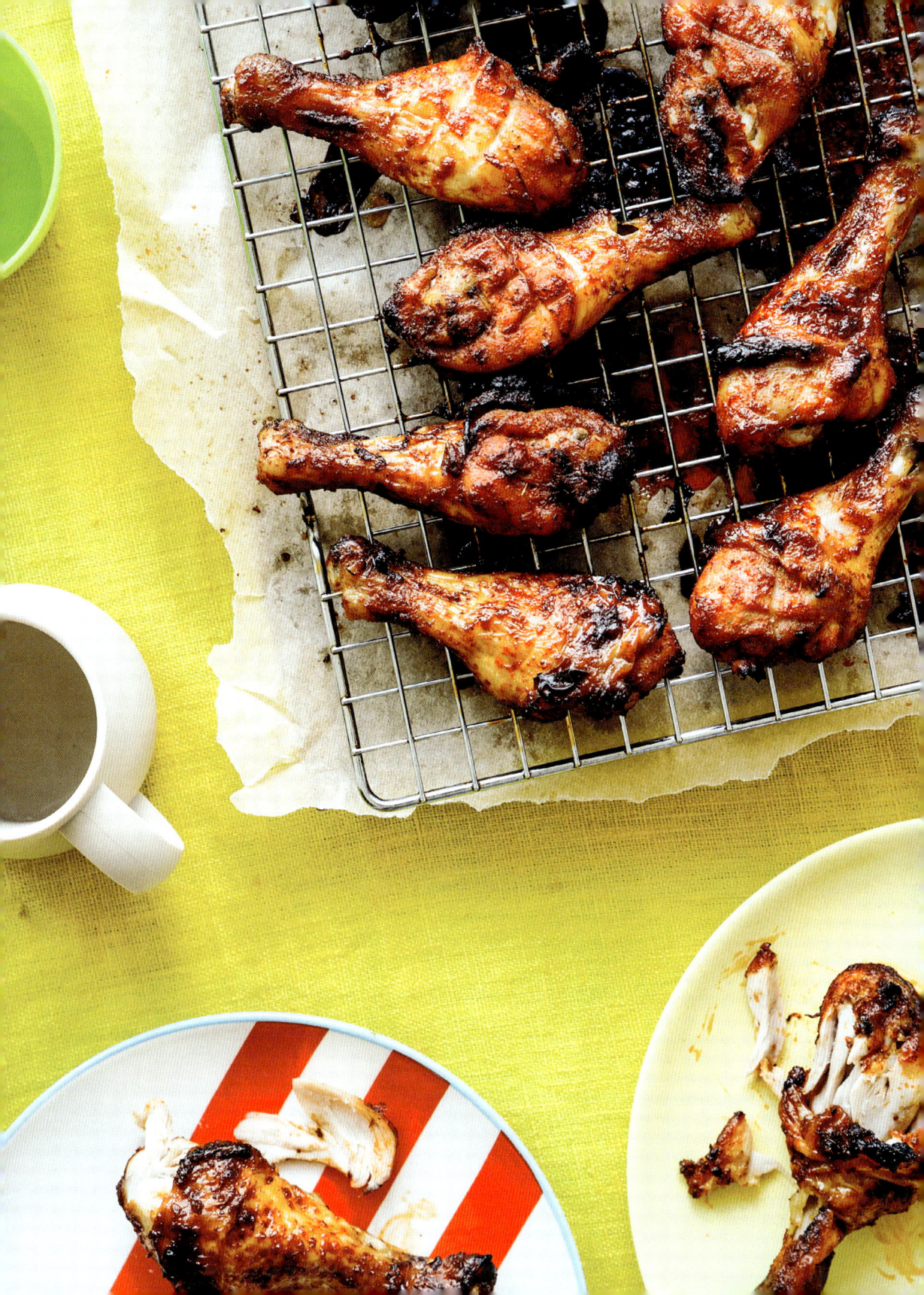

Smoky Honey Chicken Drumsticks (continued)

STORAGE & REHEATING

Store the drumsticks in an airtight container in the refrigerator for up to 3 days or freeze for up to 3 months. Thaw the frozen drumsticks overnight in the refrigerator.

To reheat, place the (thawed) chicken drumsticks on a large baking sheet lined with parchment paper and cook them at 350°F (180°C, gas mark 4, 160°C fan) for 15 to 20 minutes, or until they are heated through.

NOTES

Chicken drumsticks can be served whole at around 12 to 24 months, once you feel your toddler's eating skills have developed proficiently—just be sure to remove the pin bones and loose cartilage before serving. You may also wish to remove the skin before 24 months, as some toddlers may find the texture challenging before then. If in doubt, remove the chicken from the bone and serve shredded or in bite-size pieces.

Oven-Baked Turkey & Spinach Meatballs

I have a love–hate relationship with meatballs. I love them for the warmth and comfort they bring to the dinner table and the fact that my kids will never turn them down, but I dislike the time it takes to roll the meatballs, fry them off and then babysit them over the stove while they bubble away—not to mention the fact that the sauce almost always splatters both myself (ouch) and the kitchen walls when I remove the lid from the pot to stir them.

This recipe solves half of this problem—yes, I still have to roll the meatballs, but that's the only time-consuming part of this recipe, which I can do in advance should I need to. After that, everything goes into a large baking dish which then goes right in the oven, not to be disturbed until its ready to serve. I love it! I also love how well the turkey holds up with this method and the way it remains deliciously moist. The flavors also work very well with the spinach and parmesan. I like to serve the meatballs as meatball subs or with my Easy Garlic Noodles (page 112).

Serves: 4

Prep Time: 15 minutes

Cook Time: 45 to 50 minutes

INGREDIENTS

1 medium brown onion, finely chopped

2 garlic cloves, minced

MEATBALLS

1.1 lbs (500 g) lean ground turkey

2 cups (60 g) tightly packed baby spinach, finely chopped

1 large egg (see notes for substitution tips)

⅔ cup (65 g) finely grated parmesan or ¼ cup (60 g) nutritional yeast (nondairy option)

½ cup (30 g) panko breadcrumbs

1 tsp garlic granules or powder

2 tsp (2 g) Italian seasoning

Black pepper, to taste

METHOD

Preheat the oven to 400°F (200°C, gas mark 6, fan 180°C).

In a large baking dish, add the chopped onion and minced garlic, and spread them out into an even layer. Set aside.

In a large bowl, add the ground turkey, chopped baby spinach, egg, grated parmesan, panko breadcrumbs, garlic granules, Italian seasoning and black pepper. Using your hands, mix everything until well combined and roll the mixture into balls around 1½ to 2 inches (3 to 4 cm) in size. Add the rolled meatballs in an even layer over the chopped onion and garlic. Bake in the oven for 10 minutes.

(Continued)

MAKE-AHEAD

FREEZER FRIENDLY

SOURCE OF IRON & PROTEIN

NUTRITIOUS & DELICIOUS MAINS THAT LITTLE ONES WILL LOVE

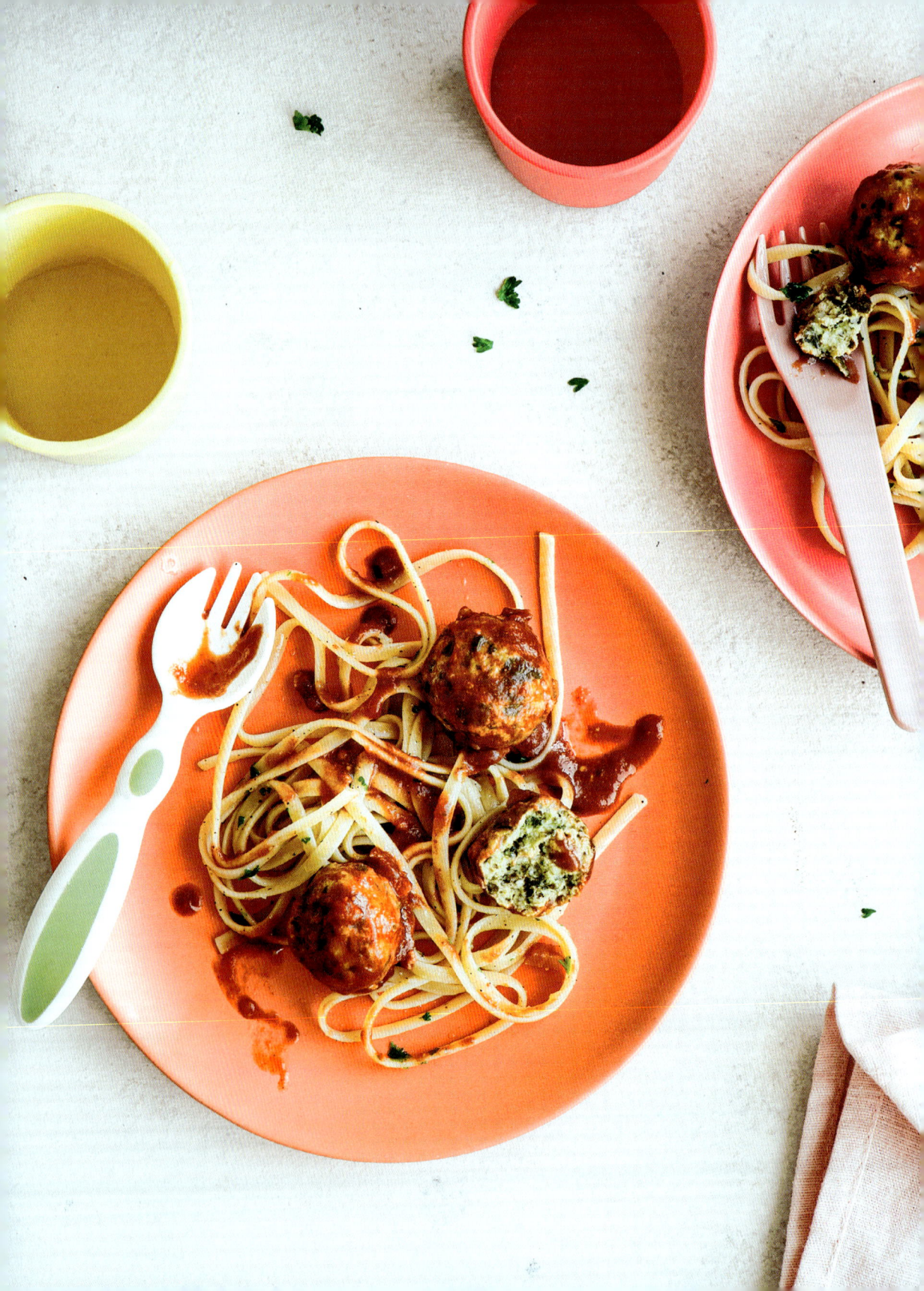

Oven-Baked Turkey & Spinach Meatballs (continued)

TOMATO SAUCE

1 cup (240 ml) beef stock

1 (15 oz [400 g]) can finely chopped tomatoes or crushed tomatoes

17.5 oz (500 g) passata or sieved tomatoes

2 tbsp (30 g) tomato paste

2 tbsp (30 ml) Worcestershire sauce

Salt and black pepper, to taste

Meanwhile, combine the beef stock, canned tomatoes, passata, tomato paste, Worcestershire sauce, salt and black pepper in a large bowl or jug and whisk until well combined. Remove the meatballs from the oven, pour over the tomato sauce mixture and gently stir everything together. Place the baking dish back in the oven and cook for 35 to 40 minutes, or until the meatballs are cooked through and sauce is bubbling and has thickened to your liking. Mix thoroughly and allow to cool sufficiently before serving.

STORAGE & REHEATING

Store in an airtight container in the refrigerator for up to 3 days. To freeze the meatballs, divide them into individual portions (if desired) and freeze them for up to 3 months. Thaw the meatballs in the refrigerator before reheating, or gently reheat them on the stove from frozen with a splash of water until fully defrosted and piping hot all the way through.

NOTES

In this recipe, the egg is used to prevent the meatballs from falling apart during cooking and serving. If you need to replace the eggs, I recommend using 2 tablespoons (30 ml) of one of the following options: tomato paste, plain yogurt of choice, buttermilk, ricotta cheese or unsweetened applesauce.

Serves:
4

Prep Time:
6 minutes

Cook Time:
35 minutes

VEGAN OPTION

SOURCE OF FIBER

Sweet Potato Mini Pizzas

First, I want to be clear that this recipe is not about trying to create a "healthy" version of pizza. We love regular pizza and eat it often, and nothing can beat the real thing! This recipe was inspired by these cute little cheese and tomato paste topped baked eggplant slices I used to make for my kids years ago—they tasted great, but I remember my toddlers being frustrated by how soft and mushy the texture of the eggplant was, which made them tricky to eat. To remedy this, I decided to try sweet potato as a base instead, as well as switching to pizza sauce, and let me tell you, this was a wonderful upgrade. It quickly became a favorite! In terms of toppings, I prefer to keep things simple here, but feel free to add in any toppings you like, and you can also speed things up by using store-bought pizza sauce.

INGREDIENTS

SWEET POTATO BASES

4 large sweet potatoes, cut into 0.4-inch (1-cm)-thick rounds

Nonstick cooking spray, as needed

Salt and black pepper, to taste

1 cup (115 g) grated mozzarella cheese or nondairy cheese of choice

Toppings of choice

PIZZA SAUCE

¼ cup (60 g) passata or strained tomatoes

2 tbsp (30 g) tomato paste

½ tsp garlic granules or powder

1 tsp dried oregano

METHOD

Preheat the oven to 400°F (200°C, gas mark 6, fan 180°C) and line two large rimmed baking sheets with parchment paper.

Arrange the sliced sweet potato in an even layer on the two baking sheets, ensuring none of them are touching. Spray generously with the nonstick cooking spray and season with some salt and black pepper. Bake in the oven for 20 minutes.

Meanwhile, in a small bowl, add all of the ingredients for the pizza sauce and mix until well combined. Set aside.

Carefully remove the baking sheets from the oven. Evenly spoon the pizza sauce on top of each sweet potato slice and top them with some mozzarella cheese and any toppings you are adding. Pop the baking sheets back into the oven and cook for 15 minutes, or until the cheese is golden and bubbling.

The sweet potato pizzas will be very hot, so be sure to give them enough time to cool off before serving.

STORAGE & REHEATING

Store in an airtight container in the refrigerator for up to 2 days. To reheat, place the sweet potato pizzas in an even layer in a baking dish and cook in the oven at 350°F (180°C, gas mark 4, fan 160°C) for 10 minutes, or until warmed through.

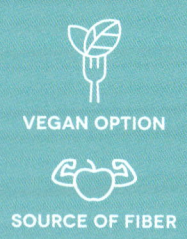

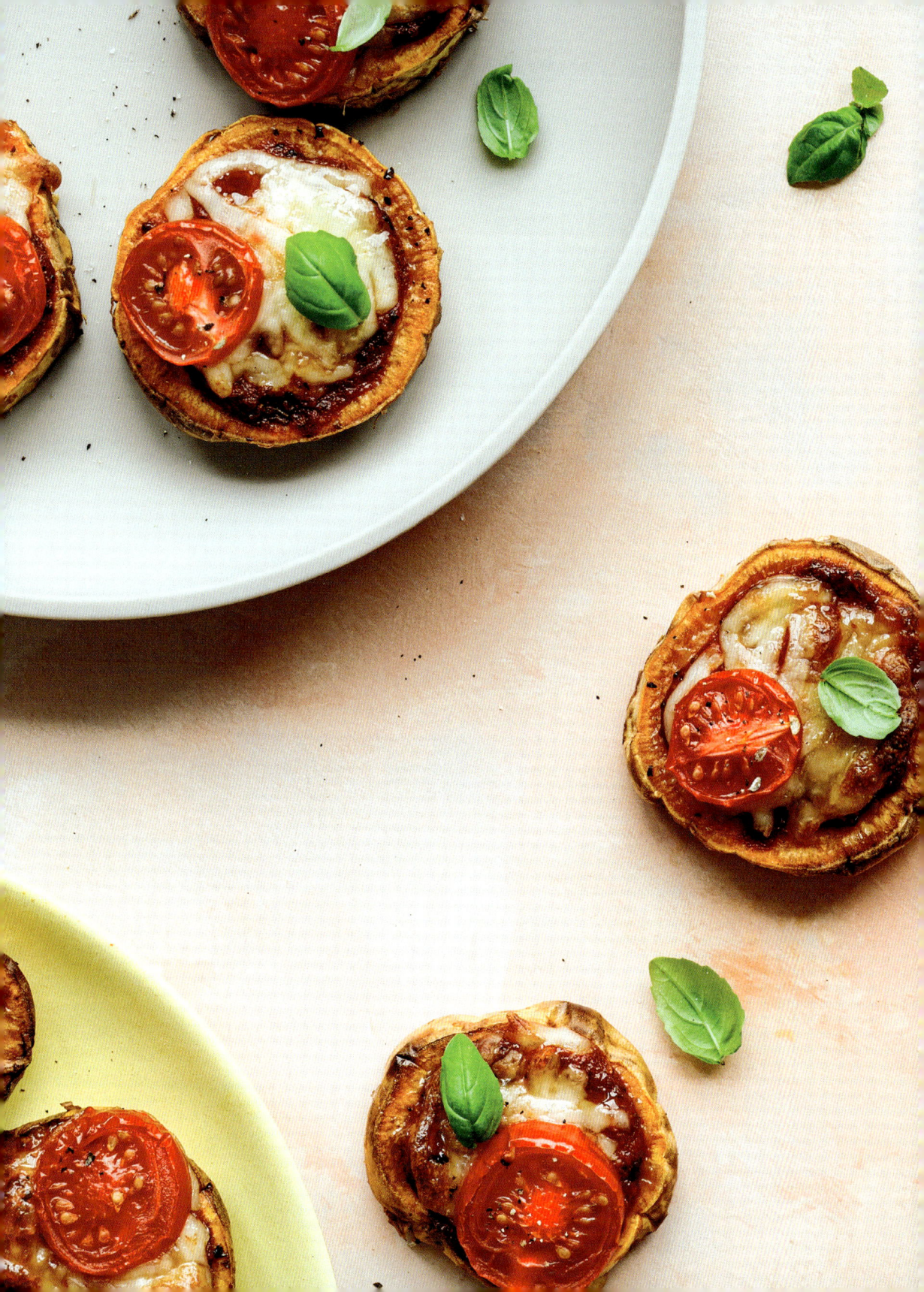

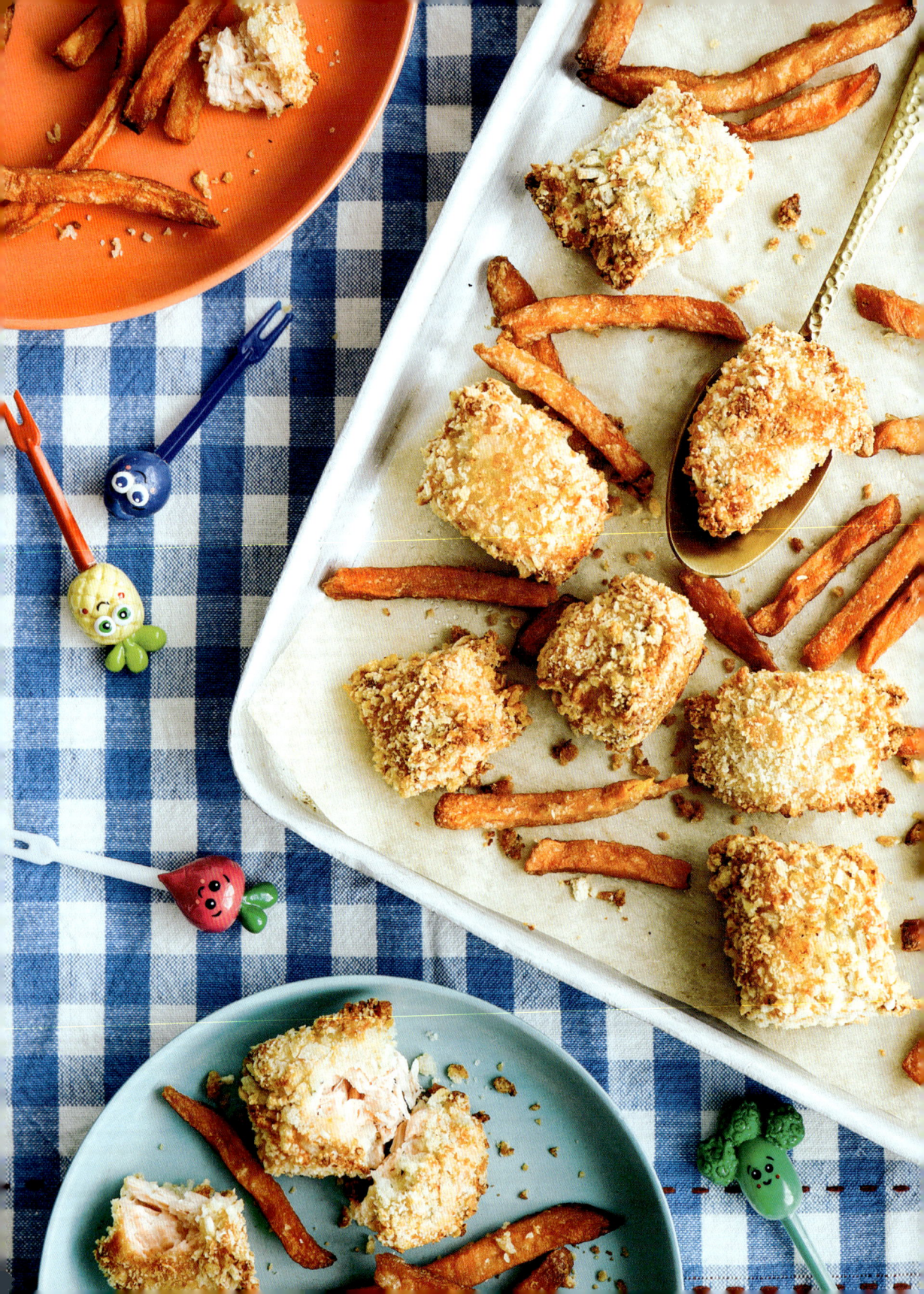

Crispy Salmon Bites

If there's one thing that I love to do, it's to take a much-loved kid's classic and make it into something that adults will also look forward to eating. Store-bought frozen fish sticks were a staple in my childhood and my kids adore them too. Even to this day, I'm partial to a fish finger and mayonnaise sandwich. But I'd be fibbing if I said, all these years later, that frozen fish sticks were something I really looked forward to eating for my dinner. Convenient, yes—but let's just say my palate has evolved over the years! These salmon bites are the perfect solution—supremely crispy and packed full of flavor from the seasonings and parmesan while still embodying their familiar appearance of beige-ness that kids just seem to flock to. Using salmon as the fish of choice means even more flavor and a nice boost of healthy fat and iron. Even my fish-hating toddler eats these with a squirt of ketchup and some fries!

Serves: 4

Prep Time: 15 minutes

Cook Time: 15 to 20 minutes

INGREDIENTS

2 large eggs

1 tsp garlic granules or powder

1 tsp onion granules or powder

1 tsp dried dill

Salt and black pepper, to taste

¼ cup (30 g) all-purpose flour

4 (4 oz [120 g]) salmon filets, cut into approximately 1.5 x 1.5 inch (4 x 4 cm) pieces

1 cup (60 g) panko breadcrumbs

½ cup (50 g) finely grated parmesan cheese or ¼ cup (60 g) nutritional yeast (nondairy option)

Nonstick cooking spray, as needed

METHOD

Preheat the oven to 400°F (200°C, gas mark 6, fan 180°C) and line a large baking sheet with parchment paper.

Crack the eggs into a medium bowl and whisk until smooth. Add the garlic granules, onion granules, dried dill, salt, black pepper and flour. Whisk the ingredients together until a smooth batter forms. Add the salmon pieces to the bowl and stir until all of the pieces are coated in the batter. Set the bowl aside.

In a shallow baking dish or bowl, mix together the breadcrumbs and parmesan. Roll one piece of salmon at a time in the breadcrumb mixture, making sure all of the sides are coated, and transfer each piece of salmon to the lined baking sheet in an even layer. (Note: If you are making these ahead of time, this is where you will freeze them—see storage and reheating notes for full instructions).

Spray the salmon bites with the nonstick cooking spray and bake them in the oven for 15 to 20 minutes, or until they are golden, crispy and fully cooked through.

(Continued)

MAKE-AHEAD

FREEZER FRIENDLY

ALLERGEN: EGG

SOURCE OF HEALTHY FATS, IRON & PROTEIN

NUTRITIOUS & DELICIOUS MAINS THAT LITTLE ONES WILL LOVE

Crispy Salmon Bites (continued)

STORAGE & REHEATING

Store leftovers in an airtight container in the refrigerator for up to 3 days or freeze for up to 3 months. If freezing the salmon bites ahead of time, arrange them in an airtight container uncooked (after coating them in the breadcrumb mixture), layering them in even layers between sheets of parchment paper and freeze for up to 3 months.

To cook the frozen salmon bites, place them on a large baking sheet lined with parchment paper and bake them at 400°F (200°C, gas mark 6, fan 180°C) for 20 to 25 minutes, or until they are golden and fully cooked through.

Hearty Mexican Chicken Quesadillas

It's no secret that I love Mexican food and it often inspires my cooking. This recipe came about from my family's love for chicken fajitas, and the fact that I wanted to be mindful of not serving them over and over, running the risk of my kids getting bored. It's very similar flavorwise, but uses a different cooking method, which makes all the difference—and the addition of melted cheese is just heavenly!

Feel free to adjust the amount of mild chili powder based on your family's preferences, and for younger toddlers you can serve the quesadilla deconstructed—this is a great option for picky eaters who may not like their food to touch. Just a heads up, the quesadillas are deceptively filling, so don't be tempted to overload your toddler's plate on first sight!

Serves: 4

Prep Time: 8 minutes

Cook Time: 25 to 30 minutes

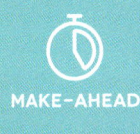

INGREDIENTS

- 2 chicken breasts, sliced into ½-inch (1-cm) strips
- ½ tsp mild chili powder
- ½ tsp smoked paprika
- ½ tsp ground cumin
- ½ tsp garlic granules or powder
- 1 tsp dried oregano
- 3 tbsp (45 ml) avocado or olive oil, divided, plus more as needed
- 1 red onion, thinly sliced
- 1 yellow pepper, thinly sliced
- 7 oz (200 g) passata or strained tomatoes
- Salt and black pepper, to taste
- 4 large tortillas of choice
- 2 cups (230 g) grated mozzarella cheese or nondairy cheese of choice, divided

METHOD

In a medium sized bowl, add the sliced chicken breast, mild chili powder, smoked paprika, ground cumin, garlic granules and oregano and mix until well combined. Allow the chicken to season for 5 minutes.

Heat a large, wide-based frying pan over medium-high heat and add 2 tablespoons (30 ml) of the oil. Once the oil is hot, add the chicken in an even layer and sear it for 2 to 3 minutes on each side, until evenly browned. Add the red onion and yellow pepper and mix to combine. Cook for 3 to 4 minutes, or until the onion and pepper begin to soften.

Add the passata and season with some salt and pepper. Cook for 2 minutes, turn the heat down to low and allow to simmer for 3 to 5 minutes, or until the chicken is fully cooked. Place a tortilla on a plate and place one-quarter of the chicken and bell pepper mixture on one side of the tortilla. Sprinkle ½ cup (58 g) of the mozzarella cheese over the chicken mixture and fold the tortilla over. Repeat this process with one more tortilla.

(Continued)

MAKE-AHEAD

SOURCE OF IRON & PROTEIN

NUTRITIOUS & DELICIOUS MAINS THAT LITTLE ONES WILL LOVE

Hearty Mexican Chicken Quesadillas (continued)

Heat a large nonstick frying pan over medium heat and add the remaining 1 tablespoon (15 ml) of oil. Once the oil is hot, carefully transfer the two folded quesadillas to the pan and cook them for 3 to 4 minutes, until the undersides are golden. Gently flip the quesadillas and cook the other sides for 3 to 4 minutes, until the quesadillas are golden and crispy and the mozzarella cheese is melted and gooey.

Repeat this process to assemble and cook the last two quesadillas, adding more oil to the pan as needed. Allow to cool sufficiently before slicing into triangles and serving.

STORAGE & REHEATING
These quesadillas are best served right after cooking, but leftovers can be stored in an airtight container in the refrigerator for up to 2 days. Reheat the quesadillas in a hot frying pan with a splash of oil.

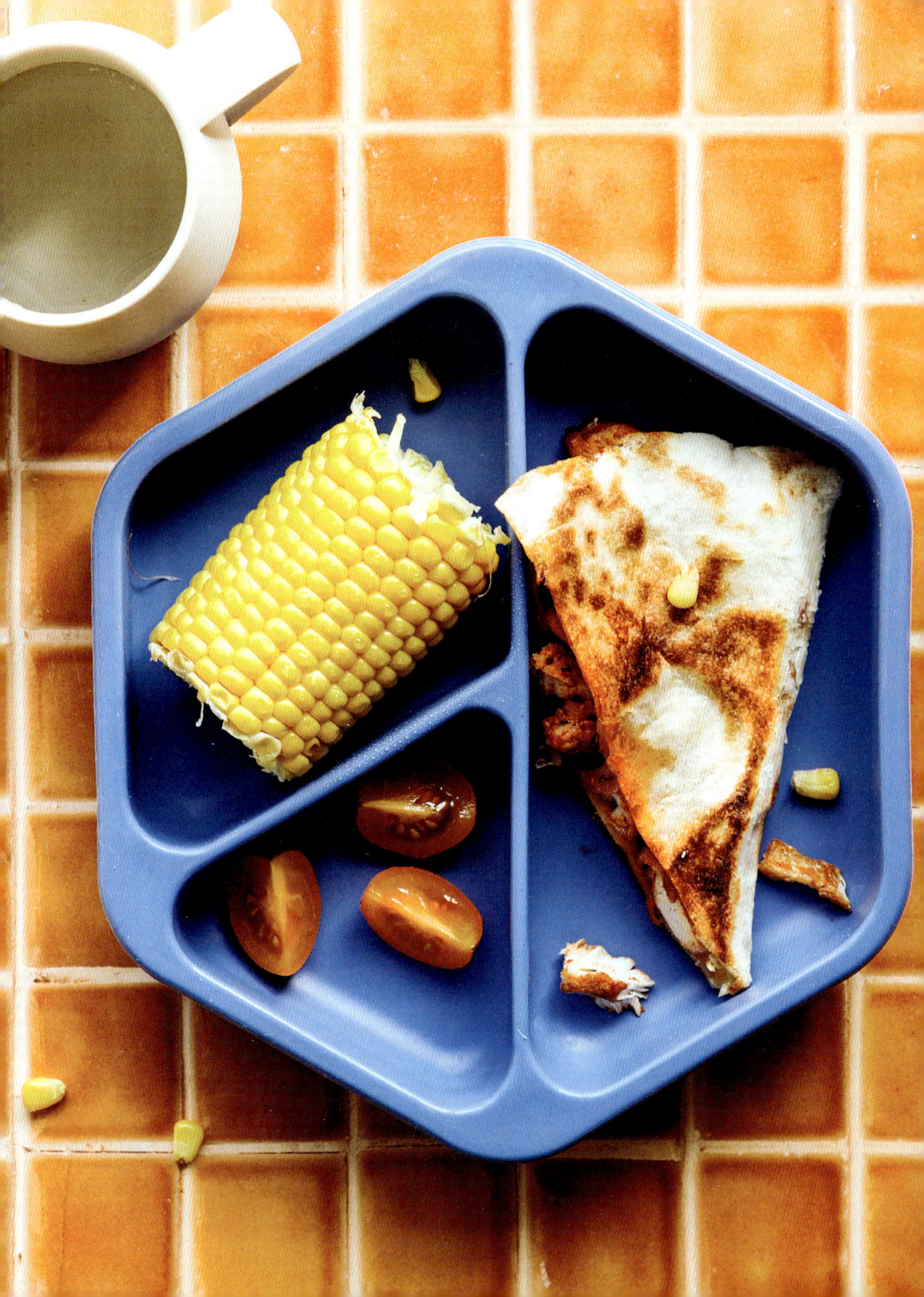

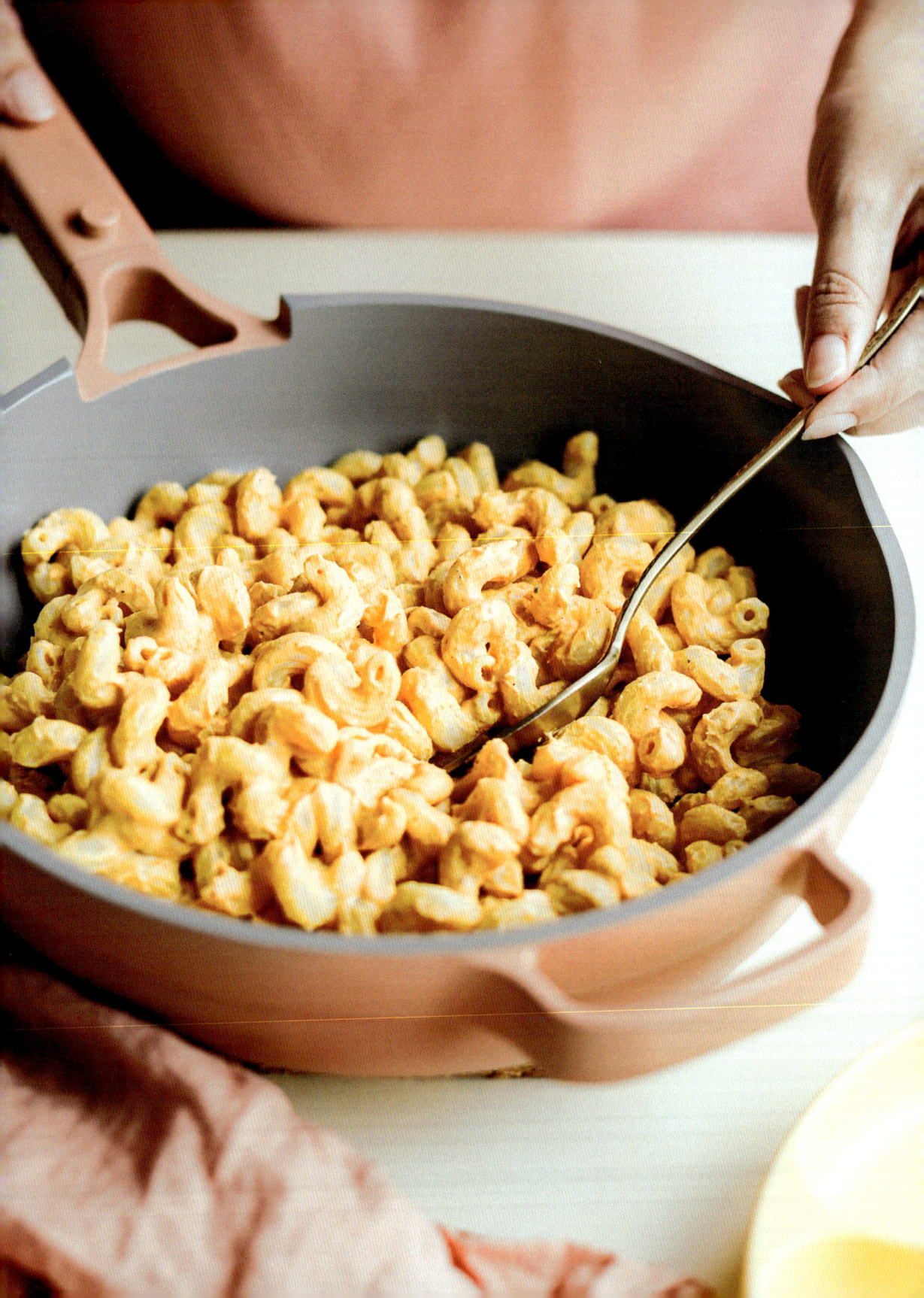

Stovetop Pumpkin Mac & Cheese

Creamy mac and cheese is an all-time kid favorite, and my kids are no strangers to this delicious classic! I first created this recipe when I needed to use up some leftover canned pumpkin, and I wasn't disappointed to find that such a simple addition would make the cheesy sauce even creamier and give it a velvet-like texture that was the epitome of comfort—not to mention, it also added such great depth of flavor. It doesn't taste of pumpkin outright, but it just gives it a certain oomph that my kids thoroughly enjoy. And of course, it has the added benefit of packing in some extra nutrients. Although that was not my initial intention, it's a great plus point!

INGREDIENTS

14 oz (400 g) chickpea or lentil pasta or pasta of choice

1 cup (250 g) canned pumpkin puree

½ cup (120 g) full-fat cream cheese

1 tsp Dijon mustard

¾ cups (80 g) grated cheddar cheese

½ tsp garlic granules or powder

½ tsp onion granules or powder

¼ tsp ground nutmeg

Salt and black pepper, to taste

METHOD

Bring a large pot of water to a boil over high heat. Add the pasta and cook it according to the package instructions.

Meanwhile, heat a medium pot over medium heat and add the pumpkin puree, cream cheese and mustard and whisk until well combined. Cook for 2 minutes, or until heated through, stirring often.

Carefully add 4 tablespoons (60 ml) of the starchy pasta water to the sauce and whisk together. Add the grated cheese, garlic granules, onion granules, ground nutmeg, salt and black pepper and mix to combine. Turn the heat down to low and cook for 2 to 3 minutes, or until the cheese has fully melted and the mixture starts to bubble, stirring all the while. Turn off the heat.

Once the pasta has cooked, drain the water and add the pasta back to the pot. Pour the cheesy pumpkin sauce over the pasta and mix until all the of the pasta is coated in the sauce. Allow to cool sufficiently before serving.

STORAGE

This dish is best served fresh; however, leftovers can be stored in an airtight container in the refrigerator for up to 2 days.

Serves: 4

Prep Time: 5 minutes

Cook Time: 15 to 20 minutes

30 READY IN 30 MINUTES OR LESS

VEGETARIAN

ALLERGEN: DAIRY

SOURCE OF IRON & PROTEIN

Serves:
4

Prep Time:
10 minutes +
30 minutes to chill

Cook Time:
20 minutes

MAKE-AHEAD

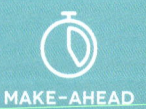

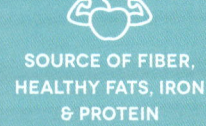

FREEZER FRIENDLY

SOURCE OF FIBER,
HEALTHY FATS, IRON
& PROTEIN

Lamb Kofta & Tzatziki Dip

Lamb has such a wonderful mellow and slightly sweet flavor and is a fantastic source of absorbable iron for toddlers, but these days it can be very pricey. My lamb koftas are a more affordable way to serve lamb to your family and they make for a great make-ahead meal for those busy evenings. Typically associated with the Middle East, lamb koftas are the perfect blend of punchy herbs and aromatic spices, which always remind me of summer and being on holiday!

This recipe is made on the stovetop but is perfect for grilling too. Feel free to add some additional shredded veggies to bulk out the kofta mixture, and you can even separate half of the kofta mixture and add some red chili flakes to heat things up for the adults. My tried and tested tzatziki recipe is the perfect companion for the koftas, and I've been making it for years, without complaint from my children. I like to stuff the koftas into fluffy flatbreads that I buy from my local bakery, topped with copious amounts of tzatziki and some crisp lettuce and chopped tomatoes. This meal is fabulous served with my Sautéed Green Beans (page 111) on the side!

INGREDIENTS

FOR THE LAMB KOFTAS

1.1 lb (500 g) ground lamb

1 small brown onion, peeled and shredded

2 garlic cloves, minced

¼ cup (15 g) panko breadcrumbs

1 tsp ground coriander

1 tsp ground cumin

1 tsp smoked paprika

¼ tsp ground cinnamon

Salt and black pepper, to taste

2 tbsp (6 g) chopped fresh mint or 1 tsp dried mint

2 tbsp (6 g) chopped fresh cilantro or 1 tsp dried cilantro leaves

2 tbsp (30 ml) avocado or olive oil, for frying

METHOD

In a large bowl, add the all the ingredients for the lamb koftas (except the avocado oil). Using your hands, gently mix everything together until all of the ingredients are well combined. Divide the mixture into 12 balls and roll them into log shapes, then gently flatten the sides of each log so that they are the same thickness from top to bottom. Transfer the lamb koftas onto a plate lined with parchment paper and refrigerate for at least 30 minutes.

While the lamb koftas are chilling, grab a small bowl and add all the ingredients for the tzatziki dip (see next page 78 for tzatziki ingredients list). Mix them together until well combined. Cover and refrigerate until needed.

Remove the lamb koftas from the refrigerator, heat a large nonstick frying pan over medium heat and add the avocado oil. Once the oil is hot, add the koftas in an even layer and cook them for 4 to 5 minutes on each side, or until well browned and cooked all the way through. Serve with the tzatziki dip plus some additional sides of your choosing (see recipe introduction for suggestions).

(Continued)

76 FEEDING TODDLERS

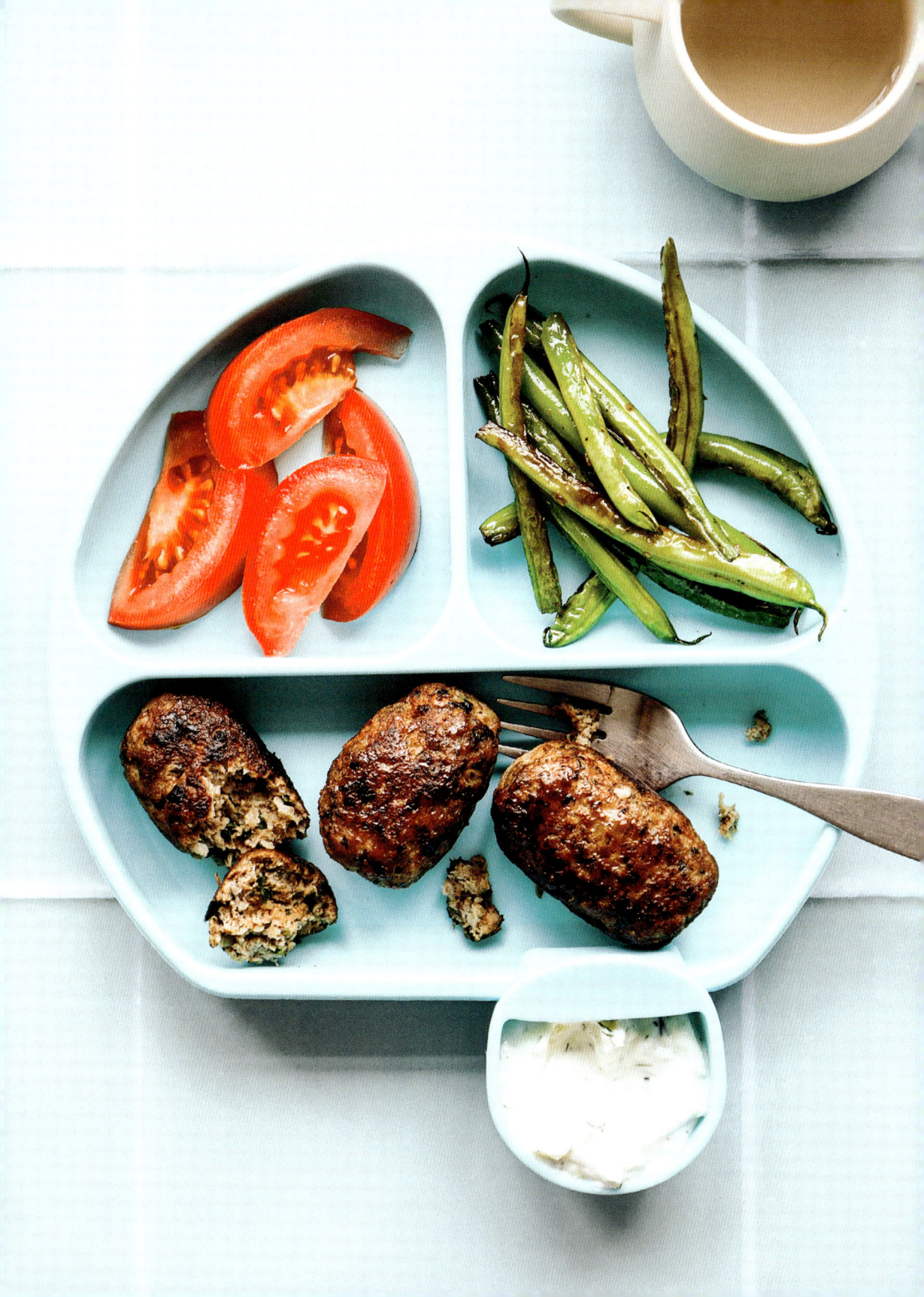

Lamb Kofta & Tzatziki Dip (continued)

FOR THE TZATZIKI

⅓ large English cucumber, deseeded and shredded

1 cup (280 g) plain Greek or natural yogurt or plain nondairy yogurt of choice

1 garlic clove, minced

2 tbsp (6 g) chopped fresh dill or 1 tsp dried dill

Juice of 1 medium lemon

Salt and black pepper, to taste

STORAGE & REHEATING

Store the cooked lamb koftas in an airtight container in the refrigerator for up to 3 days or freeze for up to 3 months. To reheat the thawed koftas, place them on a large baking sheet lined with parchment paper and cook them (covered) at 350°F (180°C, gas mark 4, fan 160°C) for 15 to 20 minutes, or until they are heated through.

Store the tzatziki in an airtight container in the refrigerator for up to 5 days, or until the yogurt expires, if earlier.

Lazy Lasagna Soup

If you're anything like me and you love lasagna but hate all the meal prep and layering that comes with it, then you will love this recipe, which takes all the wonderful parts of a lasagna and makes them into a simple, delicious and hearty soup. It might sound strange but trust me, it works! The key to getting that iconic lasagna flavor is to add a generous dollop of the cheese mix on top of the soup, which just brings everything together so perfectly. Using ground pork and ground beef together provides great depth of flavor, but feel free to substitute the pork with ground turkey or use all beef if preferred. You can also bulk up the meat sauce with some veggies if you want to pack in some extra nutrition.

Serves: 6

Prep Time: 5 minutes

Cook Time: 35 to 40 minutes

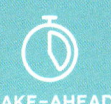

INGREDIENTS

FOR THE LASAGNA

- 0.9 lb (400 g) lean ground beef
- 0.9 lb (400 g) lean ground pork
- 2 medium brown onions, finely chopped
- 1 large red bell pepper, deseeded and finely chopped
- 4 garlic cloves, minced
- Salt and black pepper, to taste
- 1 tbsp (3 g) Italian seasoning
- 2 (15-oz [400-g]) cans finely chopped tomatoes or crushed tomatoes
- 2 cups (480 g) passata or sieved tomatoes
- 2 tbsp (30 g) tomato paste
- 4 cups (960 ml) water
- 2 cups (480 ml) beef stock
- 8 oz (230 g) Mafalda corta pasta, or pasta of choice

METHOD

Heat a large pot over medium heat, add the ground beef and ground pork and cook them for 4 to 5 minutes. As they cook, break the meat apart with a wooden spoon and mix them together until there is no pink remaining in the meat. Transfer the meat to a plate and set it aside.

Discard most of the leftover fat, leaving only a thin layer in the pot. Reduce the heat to medium. Add the onion and bell pepper and cook them for 3 minutes. Add the garlic and cook for 1 minute, until fragrant. Transfer the beef and pork back to the pot, then add some salt, black pepper and the Italian seasoning. Mix to combine, then add the canned tomatoes, passata, tomato paste, water and beef stock. Mix until everything is well combined and bring to a boil. Turn the heat down to low, cover and simmer for 10 minutes.

Turn the heat up to medium, bring to a boil and add the pasta to the pot. Cook uncovered for 15 to 20 minutes, or until the pasta is tender, stirring often.

Meanwhile, in a small bowl, mix together the ricotta, parmesan and fresh parsley until everything is well combined (see page 81 for ingredients list). To serve, ladle the soup into a bowl and top with a dollop of the cheese mixture.

(Continued)

MAKE-AHEAD

FREEZER FRIENDLY

ALLERGEN: DAIRY

SOURCE OF IRON & PROTEIN

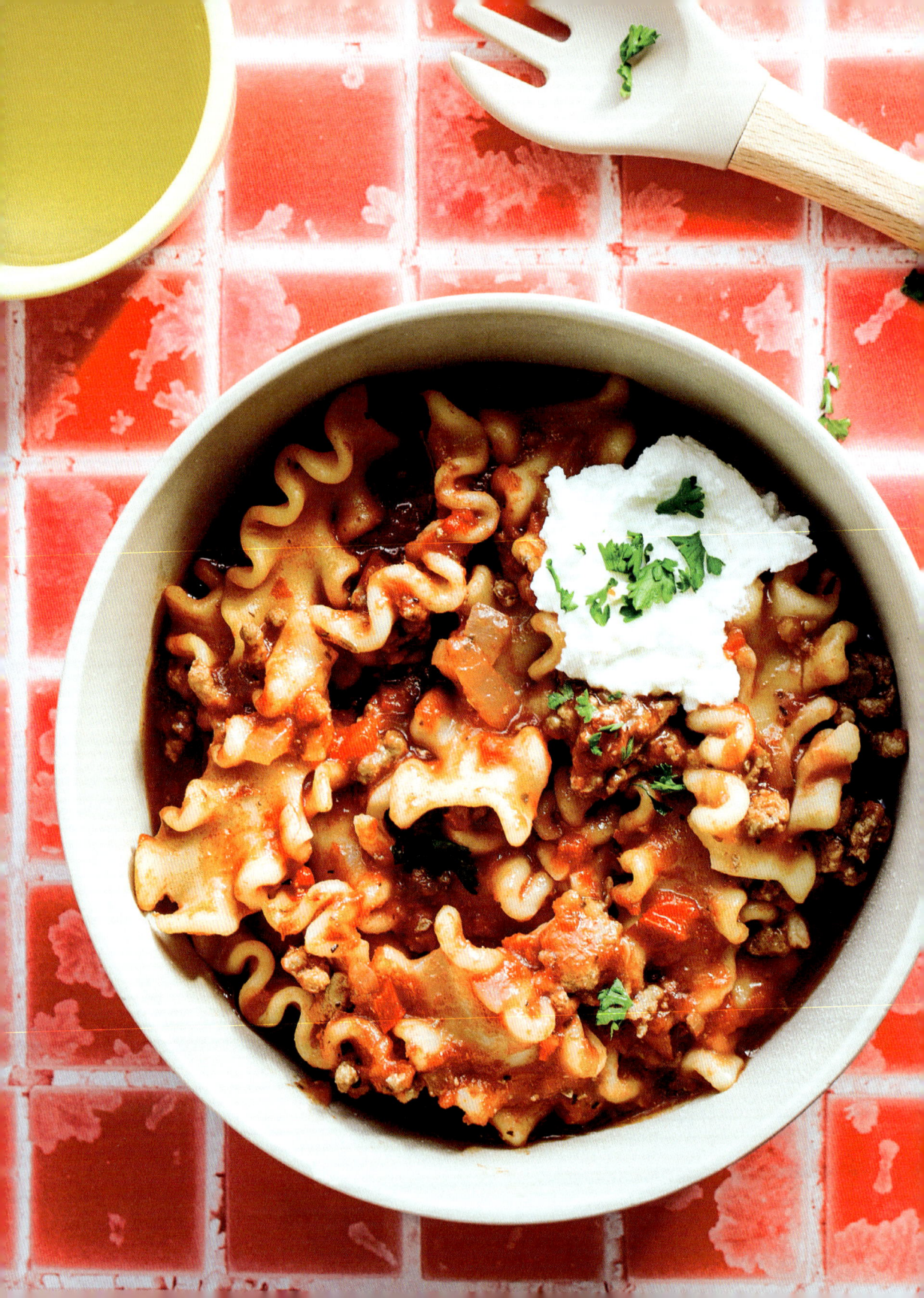

Lazy Lasagna Soup (continued)

FOR THE CHEESE MIX

¾ cup (185 g) ricotta cheese

¼ cup (25 g) finely grated parmesan

2 tbsp (6 g) chopped fresh parsley (optional)

STORAGE & REHEATING

Store the lasagna soup in an airtight container in the refrigerator for up to 3 days or freeze for up to 3 months. Reheat the thawed soup on the stove with a splash of water until warmed through.

Store the cheese mix in the refrigerator in an airtight container for up to 3 days, or until either of the cheeses expire, if earlier.

Serves:
6

Prep Time:
10 minutes

Cook Time:
50 to 55 minutes

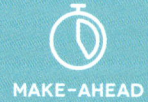

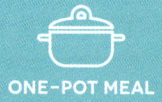

MAKE-AHEAD

ONE-POT MEAL

FREEZER FRIENDLY

VEGAN

SOURCE OF FIBER, IRON & PROTEIN

Curried Lentil & Veggie Soup

Soups are a regular feature in our home as they are such a simple, low fuss way to get some nutrients into tiny tummies. And what's more, they are made in just one pot, which will always be my favorite kind of meal—the less washing up the better! This iron- and protein-rich recipe is absolutely bursting with goodness and is another Zayne's Plate classic that I just couldn't leave out of this cookbook. It has saved me so many times when my toddler was teething, and whenever they were going through a veggie-hating phase, I would just blend it all up and watch them go to town. The mild notes of curry add extra warmth, making this soup a wonderful cold weather charmer—but in its true versatility, it's light and fresh enough for a warm sunny day too. This soup is a firm favorite with both the adults and children in my family.

INGREDIENTS

2 tbsp (30 ml) avocado or olive oil, for frying

1 large brown onion, finely chopped

2 garlic cloves, minced

2 tsp (4 g) ground cumin

1 tsp mild curry powder

1 tsp dried thyme

1 small butternut squash, peeled, deseeded and cut into 1-inch (2.5-cm) chunks

2 large carrots, peeled and cut into ½-inch (1-cm) chunks

1 cup (190 g) dried brown or green lentils, rinsed

2 (15-oz [400-g]) cans chopped tomatoes

6 cups (1.4 L) vegetable stock

Salt and black pepper, to taste

2 cups (135 g) loosely packed curly kale, tough ribs removed

METHOD

Heat a large pot over medium heat and add the avocado oil. Once the oil is hot, add the chopped onion and sauté for 3 minutes, stirring often. Add the minced garlic, ground cumin, curry powder and dried thyme and mix to combine. Cook for 1 minute until fragrant.

Add the butternut squash, carrots and brown lentils to the pot and mix well. Add the canned tomatoes, vegetable stock, salt and black pepper and give everything a good mix. Bring to a boil, turn the heat down to low and cover. Cook for 35 to 40 minutes, or until both the butternut squash and carrots are fork tender. Be sure to give it a stir once or twice while it cooks.

Remove the lid and carefully spoon three ladles of the soup into a blender. Blend until smooth, then add the blended mixture back to the soup. Mix until well combined.

Add the kale and mix to combine. Cook for 5 minutes, or until the kale is wilted and softly cooked. Serve the soup as is, or you can blend it up before serving.

STORAGE & REHEATING

Store the cooled soup in an airtight container in the refrigerator for up to 3 days. To freeze, divide the soup into individual portions (if desired) and freeze for up to 3 months. Defrost the soup overnight in the refrigerator before reheating on the stove. Alternatively, you can reheat the soup from frozen on the stove with a splash of water, gently breaking it up with a spoon as it warms through.

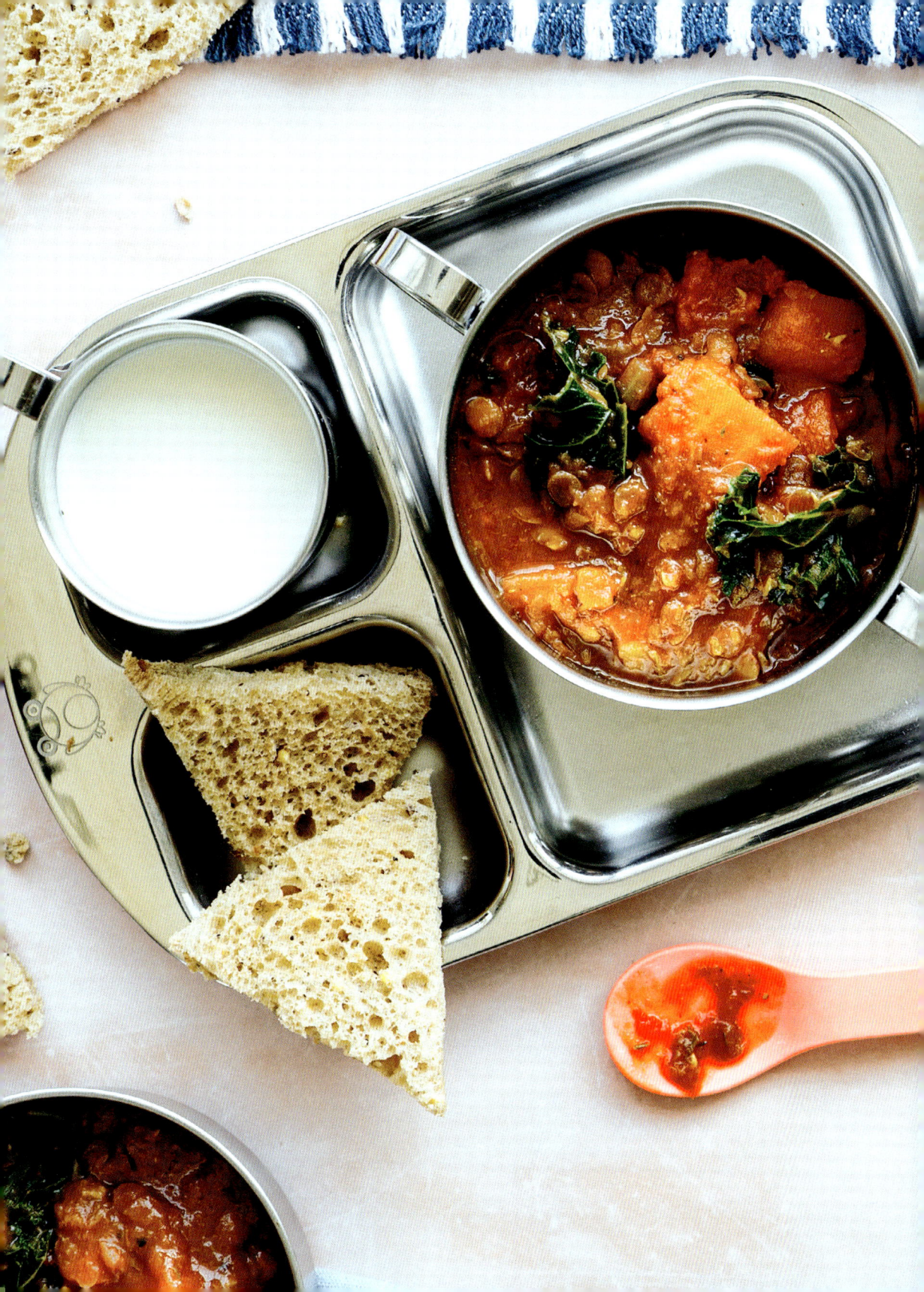

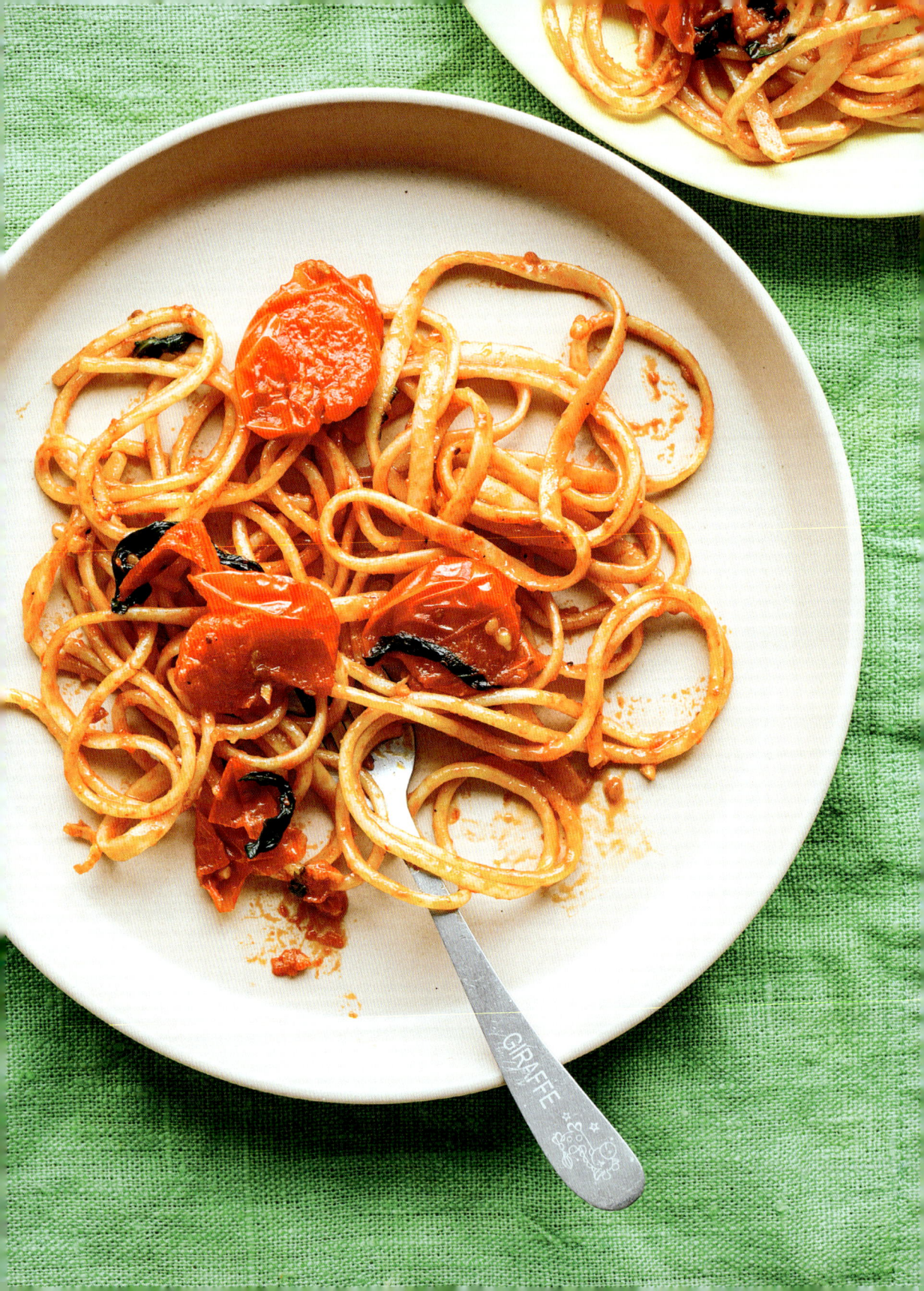

Speedy Cherry Tomato Spaghetti

I first started making this pasta dish for my youngest toddler and me as a quick lunch option during the week when everyone else was at work or school. I made it often, as I could always count on finding a box of tomatoes hiding at the back of the fridge! It gradually crept into my dinner rotation because of the sheer easiness of the recipe, and the fact that the fresh, zingy flavors were appealing to a mature palate without being too overpowering for my younger kids. I ramped up the flavor and richness by adding some butter and parmesan, but the real difference was made by switching from dried basil to fresh—I just love the pungent sweetness and inoffensive pepperiness it gives to the dish!

Serves: 4

Prep Time: 5 minutes

Cook Time: 15 to 20 minutes

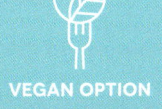

INGREDIENTS

14 oz (400 g) spaghetti or pasta of choice (see notes)

2 tbsp (30 ml) avocado or olive oil

3 cups (450 g) cherry or grape tomatoes

Salt and black pepper, to taste

4 cloves garlic, minced

2 tbsp (30 g) tomato paste

1 cup (25 g) fresh basil, roughly chopped

2 tsp (4 g) lemon zest

2 tbsp (30 g) unsalted butter or nondairy butter of choice

½ cup (50 g) freshly grated parmesan cheese or ¼ cup (60 g) nutritional yeast (nondairy option), plus more as needed, or more or less to taste

METHOD

Bring a large pot of water to a boil over high heat. Meanwhile, gather your other ingredients together. Once the water is boiled, add the spaghetti and cook it for 2 minutes less than the package instructions.

Meanwhile, heat a large nonstick, wide-based pan over medium heat and add the avocado oil. Once the oil is hot, add the cherry tomatoes, salt and pepper and cook for 3 minutes, stirring often. Add the minced garlic and cook for another 3 minutes, or until the tomatoes start to become soft.

Using the back of a spoon, gently press on the tomatoes to flatten them until they burst and release their juices. Add the tomato paste, basil and lemon zest and mix well. Cook for 2 minutes, stirring often.

Before you drain the pasta, reserve a cup (240 ml) of the starchy pasta water and add ¼ cup (60 ml) of the pasta water into the pan with the tomatoes to create a sauce—you can add more depending on how saucy you would like the end result to be. Add the butter and stir the sauce until it has melted.

Drain the pasta and add it straight into the pan with the tomatoes. Turn the heat down to low and cook for 2 minutes to marinate the flavors and finish cooking the pasta. Add the parmesan and mix through until everything is well combined. Serve with another sprinkling of grated parmesan if desired.

STORAGE

The pasta is best served freshly cooked, but leftovers can be stored in the refrigerator in an airtight container for up to 2 days.

NOTES

For added iron, choose chickpea or lentil pasta.

30 READY IN 30 MINUTES OR LESS

VEGAN OPTION

Serves:
Makes 10 to 12 fritters

Prep Time:
10 minutes

Cook Time:
6 to 8 minutes

- READY IN 30 MINUTES OR LESS
- MAKE-AHEAD
- FREEZER FRIENDLY
- LUNCHBOX FRIENDLY
- ALLERGEN: EGG & SHELLFISH
- SOURCE OF IRON & PROTEIN

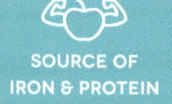

Shrimp Cakes

Shrimp has always been popular in our house—my kids love its mild, buttery, sweet flavor and it is arguably one of the less "fishy" tasting seafood options. But one thing about shrimp—it's expensive! And having a large family means I'm always trying to find ways to make it a more affordable option, and this recipe allows for just that—a little goes a long way! These fritters are like a heartier version of shrimp toast, but with a punchier and fresher flavor, and they are a match made in heaven with my creamy Lemon Garlic Dip (page 116).

INGREDIENTS

- ½ lb (225 g) raw shrimp or prawns, peeled and deveined
- 2 scallions (white and green parts), roughly chopped
- 2 large eggs
- Salt and black pepper, to taste
- 1 tsp Old Bay® Seasoning or smoked paprika
- 1 garlic clove, minced
- ¾ cup (40 g) panko breadcrumbs
- ⅓ cup (40 g) all-purpose flour or flour of choice
- ¼ cup (60 ml) avocado oil or high-heat oil of choice, for shallow frying
- Lemon Garlic Dip, for dipping (optional, page 116)

METHOD

In a food processor, add the shrimp and scallions and gently pulse until roughly chopped, being careful not to over process them into a paste.

Transfer the mixture into a large bowl and add the eggs, salt, black pepper, Old Bay® Seasoning, minced garlic, panko breadcrumbs and flour and mix until all the ingredients are well combined and you have a thick batter.

Heat a large nonstick frying pan over medium heat and add the avocado oil. Once the oil is hot, spoon 2-tablespoon (30-g) dollops of the batter to the frying pan and gently flatten them out with the back of the spoon.

Without crowding the pan, fry the fritters for 3 to 4 minutes on each side, or until they are golden and crispy and the shrimp on the inside is opaque and lightly pink in color. Transfer the fritters to a layer of paper towels to drain. Depending on the size of your pan, you may have to do this in batches. Allow the fritters to cool sufficiently and then serve them with the dip on the side, if using.

STORAGE & REHEATING

Store the fritters in an airtight container in the refrigerator for up to 3 days. To freeze, stack the fritt-ers between sheets of parchment paper in a freezer bag and freeze them for up to 3 months. Thaw the fritters in the refrigerator before reheating uncovered in the oven at 400°F (200°C, gas mark 6, 180°C fan) for around 10 minutes, or until crispy and warmed through.

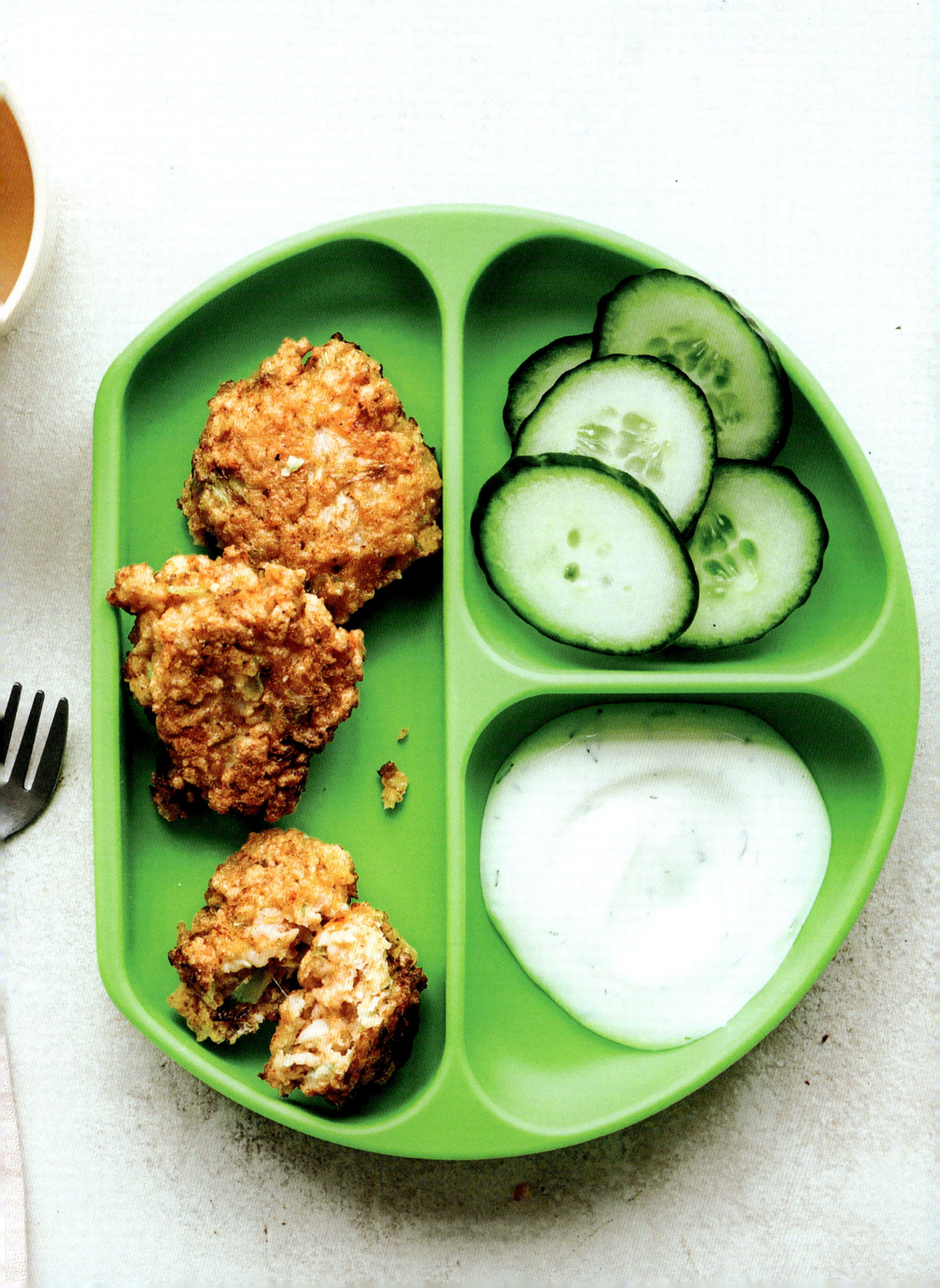

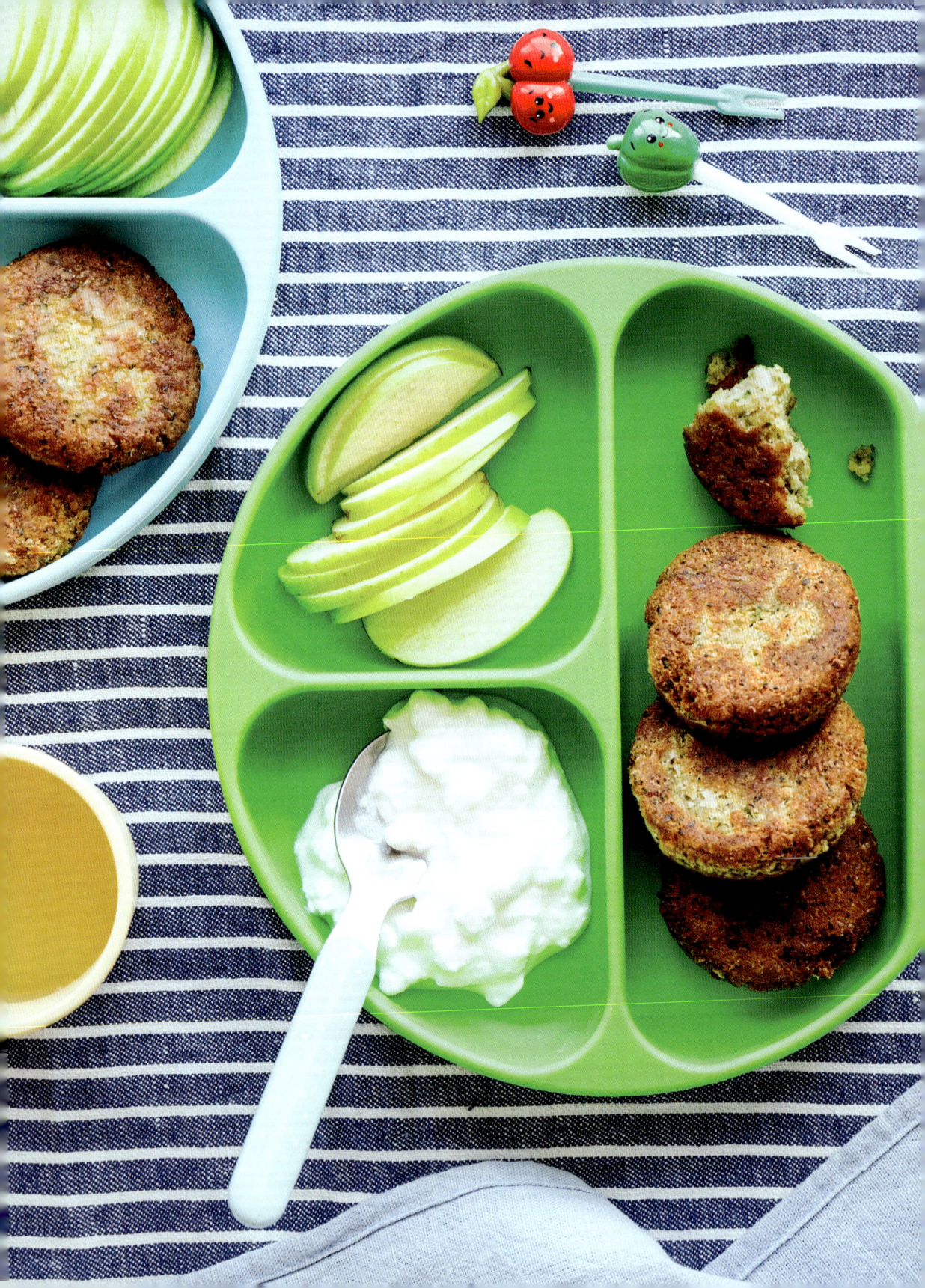

Falafel Patties

These falafel patties are not only budget friendly, they're also a great plant-based source of iron and packed with fragrant spices, giving them a gorgeously subtle yet warming flavor. And I love the texture, which is soft on the inside and crunchy on the outside—just perfection! I prefer to make falafels into mini patty shapes rather than balls because they are quicker to fry and require less babysitting at the stovetop. They also freeze well, so I recommend keeping a batch in the freezer for easy lunch and snack options.

Serves: Makes 10 to 12 patties

Prep Time: 10 minutes

Cook Time: 4 to 8 minutes

INGREDIENTS

1 (14-oz [400-g]) can chickpeas, drained and rinsed

2 scallions, roughly chopped

2 garlic cloves, peeled

¼ cup (15 g) fresh parsley

1 tsp ground cumin

1 tsp ground coriander

2 tbsp (15 g) all-purpose flour or flour of choice, plus more as needed

Salt and black pepper, taste

2 tbsp (30 ml) avocado oil or other high-heat oil, for frying

METHOD

In a food processor, add the chickpeas, scallions, garlic, parsley, ground cumin, ground coriander, flour, salt and black pepper. Blend the ingredients on high speed for 30 seconds. Remove the blender lid, scrape down the sides and then blend again in 30-second intervals until you have what looks like a moist crumbly mixture—don't be alarmed by this, the mixture will still mold into patty shapes.

Mold the mixture into patties using 2 tablespoons (30 g) of the mixture for each patty.

Heat a large nonstick frying pan over medium heat and add the oil. Once the oil is hot, add the falafel patties and cook them for 2 to 4 minutes on each side, or until they are golden brown and crispy. Transfer the falafel patties to a layer of paper towels to drain.

STORAGE & REHEATING

Store the patties in an airtight container in the refrigerator for up to 3 days. To freeze, stack the patties between sheets of parchment paper in a sealed freezer bag and freeze them for up to 3 months. Thaw the patties in the refrigerator or at room temperature before reheating in the oven at 400°F (200°C, gas mark 6, 180°C fan) for 10 minutes, or until warmed through. Alternatively, you can thaw and reheat the patties in the microwave on the high setting in 30-second intervals until fully warmed through.

30 READY IN 30 MINUTES OR LESS

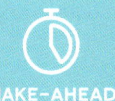

MAKE-AHEAD

FREEZER FRIENDLY

LUNCHBOX FRIENDLY

VEGAN

SOURCE OF FIBER, HEALTHY FATS, IRON & PROTEIN

Serves: 2

Prep Time: 2 minutes

Cook Time: 8 minutes

READY IN 30 MINUTES OR LESS

MAKE-AHEAD

VEGETARIAN

ALLERGEN: EGG & PEANUTS

SOURCE OF IRON & PROTEIN

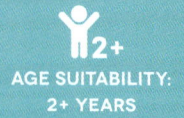

AGE SUITABILITY: 2+ YEARS

10-Minute Peanut Noodles

Most kids love pasta and peanut butter, so why not introduce them to this classic dressing combination that is super speedy to whip up and effortlessly tasty! I love that the sauce is creamy yet tangy, with a just hint of citrusy flavor. And if you want to add some veggies to the finished dish, bean sprouts, julienned carrots and julienned cucumber work perfectly. By the way, I don't recommend omitting the honey here, so with this in mind, you may wish to wait until closer to age 2 to serve this to your toddler regularly (in line with current guidance for introducing added sugars at around age 2), although a serving here and there is okay (see additional note on honey below).

INGREDIENTS

- 4.5 oz (125 g) medium egg noodles or noodles of your choice (see notes)
- 1 tbsp (15 ml) sesame oil
- 1 tbsp (15 ml) clear runny honey (see notes)
- 1 tbsp (15 ml) soy sauce
- ½ tbsp (7 ml) rice vinegar
- Small squeeze of lime
- 2 tsp (5 g) smooth peanut butter
- ½ garlic clove, minced, or more or less to taste (see notes)
- Black pepper, to taste
- 1 tsp sesame seeds (optional)

METHOD

Bring a large pot of water to a boil over high heat. Once the water is boiling, add the egg noodles and cook them according to the package instructions.

Meanwhile, add the sesame oil, honey, soy sauce, rice vinegar, lime juice, peanut butter, garlic and black pepper to a small bowl and whisk until smooth.

Once the egg noodles are cooked, drain them and add them back to the pan. Pour the peanut sauce over the noodles and mix until well combined. Distribute the peanut noodles into bowls and garnish with the sesame seeds (if using) before serving.

STORAGE & REHEATING

Store the sauce in an airtight container in the refrigerator for up to 3 days. Mix well before serving cold or reheat on the stove with a splash of water.

NOTES

If your toddler has an egg allergy, you can use any noodles of your choosing, just be aware that this may add to the total cooking time.

Honey should never be given to babies under 12 months, even when cooked. This is due to the risk of infant botulism.

If your toddler is still learning to like the flavor of raw garlic, you can switch it out for garlic granules or powder.

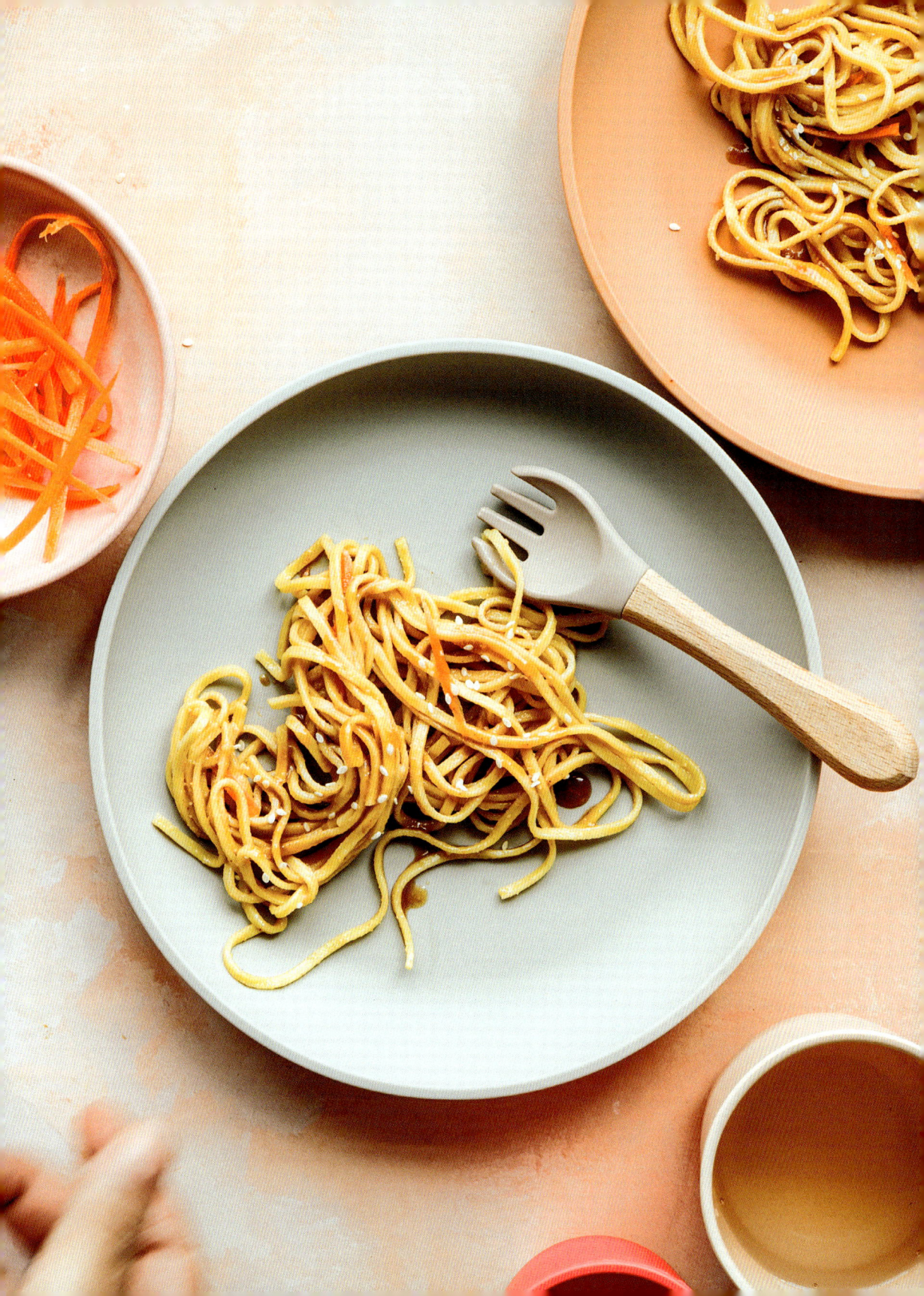

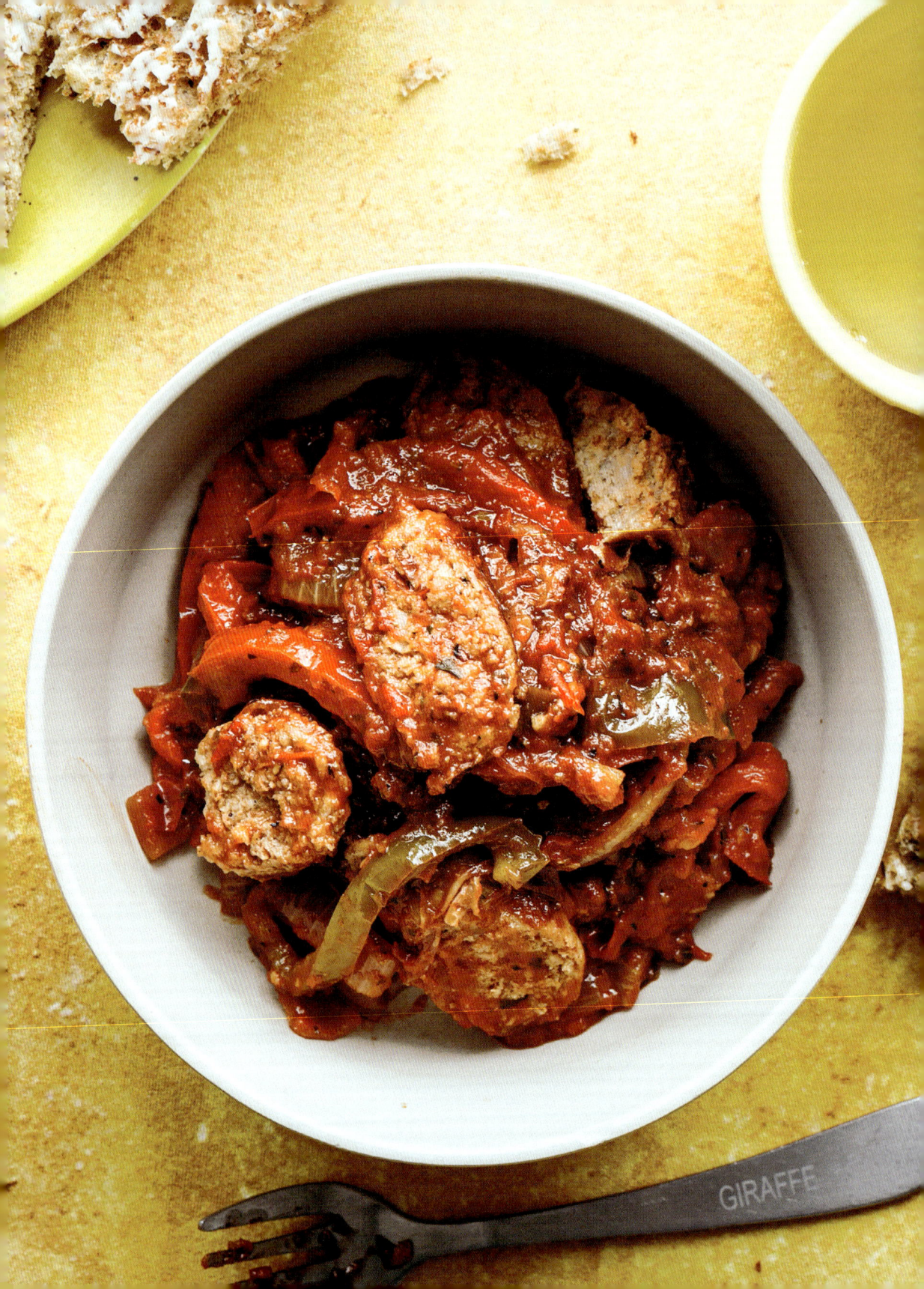

Quick-Cook Sausage & Pepper Stew

I've been making variations of fried sausage with peppers for years, typically for breakfast. I decided to add some tinned tomatoes to make a sauce, and it instantly became a super quick and easy dinner favorite. The rich, lightly spiced tomatoey flavors are reminiscent of egg shakshuka, but of course with hearty sausages instead of eggs. I generally serve it with either toast for breakfast, my Eggy Bread Rolls (page 119) for lunch or baked sweet potatoes for dinner. I have even served it over pasta with a sprinkling of cheese, which was delicious!

Serves: 4

Prep Time: 5 minutes

Cook Time: 30 minutes

INGREDIENTS

2 tbsp (30 ml) avocado or olive oil

8 standard-sized raw sausages

1 red bell pepper, thinly sliced

1 green bell pepper, thinly sliced

1 large brown onion, peeled and thinly sliced

4 garlic cloves, minced

1 tsp oregano

1 tsp smoked paprika

Salt and black pepper, to taste

1 (15-oz [400-g]) can crushed or finely chopped tomatoes

1 tbsp (15 g) tomato paste

1 tbsp (15 ml) Worcestershire sauce

METHOD

Heat a large frying pan over medium-high heat and add the avocado oil. Once the oil is hot, add the sausages in an even layer and sear them for 2 minutes on all sides, or until they are evenly browned. Remove them from the pan and set aside.

Turn the heat down to medium and add the sliced bell peppers and onion to the pan. Give them a mix and cook for 3 to 4 minutes, or until they begin to soften. Meanwhile, slice the sausages at an angle (see notes) and return them to the pan. Add the minced garlic to the pan and cook for 1 minute, then add the oregano, smoked paprika, salt and black pepper. Mix until everything is well combined and cook for 2 more minutes.

Add the canned tomatoes, tomato paste and Worcestershire sauce and mix to combine. Bring to a boil, then turn the heat down to low, cover and simmer for 10 minutes, stirring halfway through. Allow to cool sufficiently before serving.

STORAGE & REHEATING

Store the cooled stew in an airtight container in the refrigerator for up to 3 days. To freeze, divide the stew into individual portions (if desired) and freeze for up to 3 months. Defrost the stew overnight in the refrigerator before reheating on the stove with a splash of water. Alternatively, you can reheat the stew from frozen on the stove over low heat with a splash of water, gently breaking it up with a spoon as it warms through.

NOTES

The sausages are sliced at an angle to avoid serving them in perfectly round coin shapes, which are a choking hazard for kids under 4 years old. You can also cut them in half-moon shapes if desired.

MAKE-AHEAD

FREEZER FRIENDLY

SOURCE OF IRON & PROTEIN

NUTRITIOUS & DELICIOUS MAINS THAT LITTLE ONES WILL LOVE

Serves:
Makes 4 sandwiches

Prep Time:
5 minutes

Cook Time:
8 minutes +
1 hour to chill

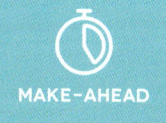

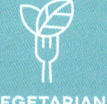

MAKE-AHEAD

LUNCHBOX FRIENDLY

VEGETARIAN

ALLERGEN: EGG

SOURCE OF
HEALTHY FATS, IRON
& PROTEIN

Avocado Egg Salad

Egg salad is a well-loved sandwich filler, and this recipe is a great twist on this kid-friendly classic. Adding mashed avocado to the mix not only adds a hearty boost of healthy fats, it also adds another layer of velvety creaminess without using a ton of mayonnaise. If you'd rather not use mayonnaise at all, you can sub it for Greek yogurt, but I personally think that it's the mayonnaise that gives egg salad such great depth of flavor, so I like to add at least **some** to the mix. This recipe comes together in one bowl in mere minutes, is budget friendly and can be made ahead of time, so if you find lunches to be a struggle, this is the recipe for you!

INGREDIENTS

4 large eggs

2 tbsp (30 ml) full-fat mayonnaise or full-fat plain Greek yogurt, plus more to taste

¼ cup (60 g) mashed avocado

½ tsp Dijon mustard

1 tsp freshly squeezed lemon juice

Salt and black pepper, to taste

METHOD

Bring a medium pot of water to a boil over high heat. Once the water reaches a rolling boil, add the eggs and cook them for 8 minutes. Once cooked, drain the eggs and place them into a bowl of ice water. Set aside to cool.

Meanwhile, in a medium bowl, add the mayonnaise, mashed avocado, Dijon mustard, lemon juice, salt and black pepper. Mix until well combined,

Peel and discard the shell from the cooled boiled eggs and chop the eggs finely. Add the chopped eggs to the mayonnaise and avocado mixture and gently mix to combine. Chill in the refrigerator for at least an hour before serving.

STORAGE

Store leftovers in an airtight container in the refrigerator for up to 3 days.

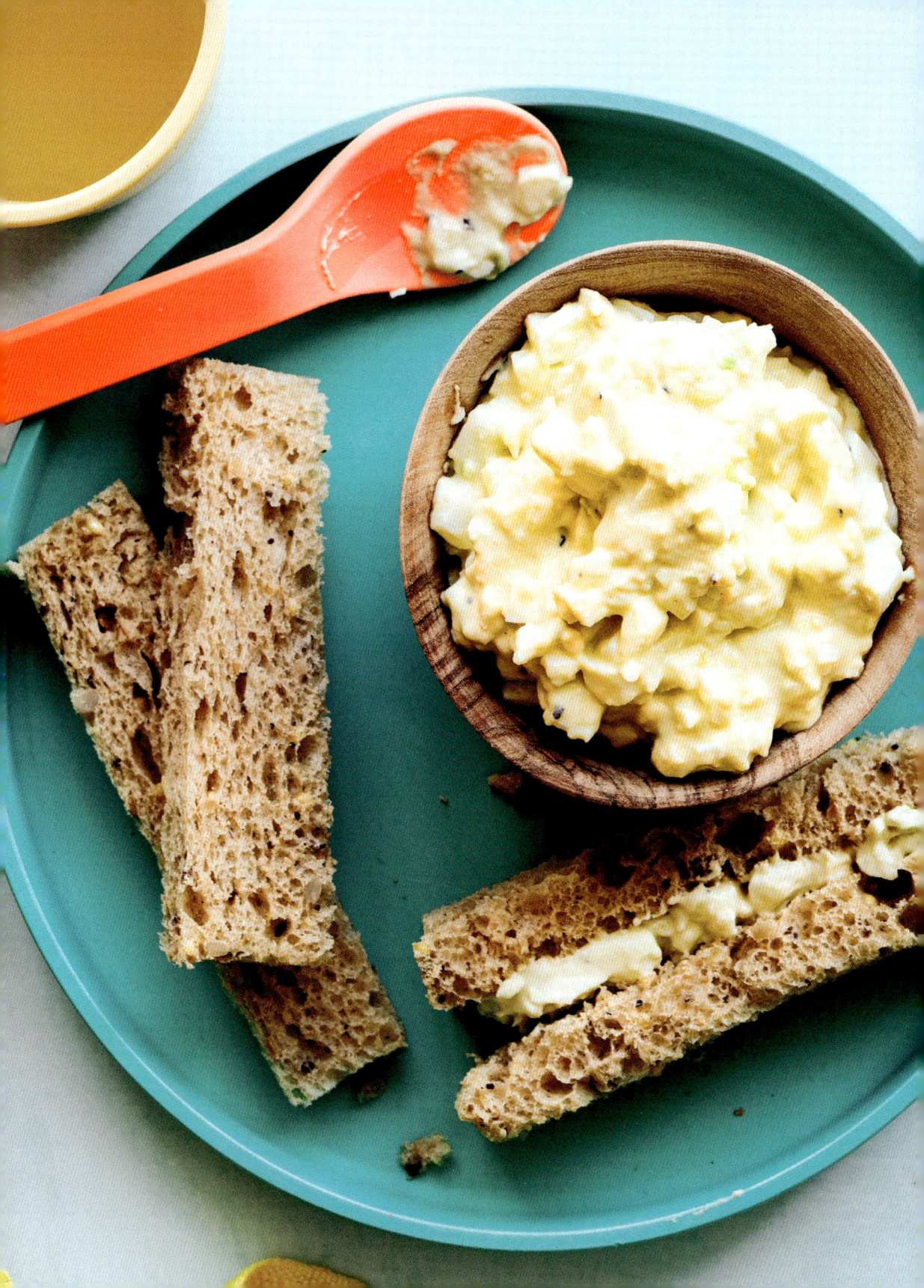

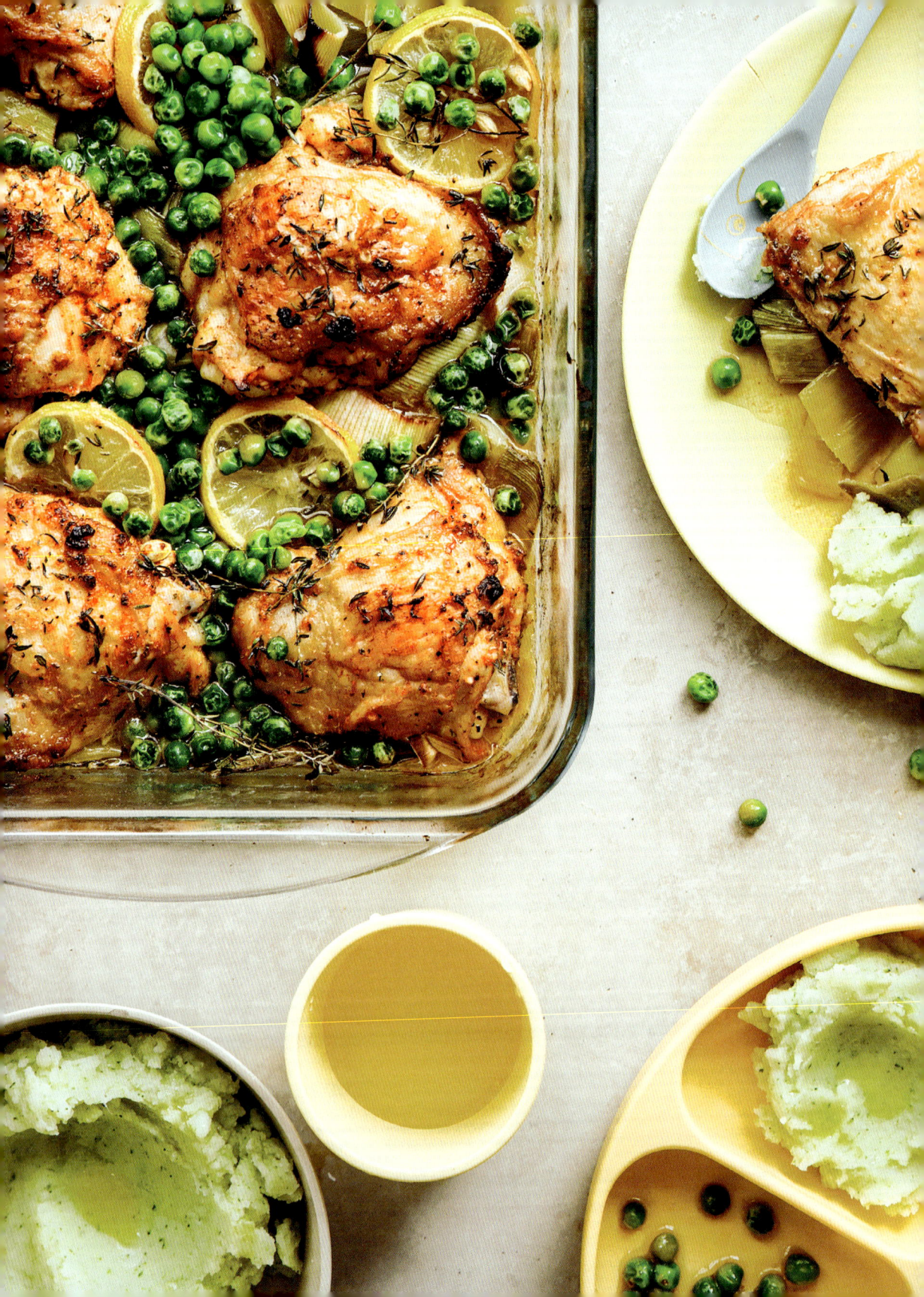

Lemony Chicken & Leek Sheet Pan

Sheet pan meals have always been my jam, and I almost always reserve them for those weeknights when I know I'll be short on time and will need something I can just dump in the oven and forget about so that the children are tended to and fed. I am in love with the way the flavors in this dish mingle and merge while cooking in the oven—a true flavor explosion that really helps to get toddlers used to punchy flavors in an unintimidating way. My favorite part is the lemony leek-infused juices that are left over in the baking dish after cooking, which I use to spoon over the chicken after serving. I like to pair this with my Parmesan Crusted Roasties (page 115), which is another dump-and-run sheet pan offering. However, if you have more hands-on time, you can also serve it with my delicious Broccoli Mashed Potatoes (page 120).

Serves: 4

Prep Time: 10 minutes

Cook Time: 45 minutes

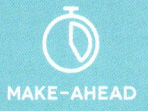

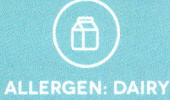

INGREDIENTS

8 chicken thighs, bone in and excess skin trimmed

4 garlic cloves, minced

2 tsp (4 g) chicken or poultry seasoning

Salt and black pepper, to taste

Juice of 1 lemon

1 large leek

1 lemon, sliced

½ cup (120 ml) hot chicken stock

¼ cup (60 ml) melted unsalted butter

2 tbsp (4 g) fresh thyme leaves or 2 tsp (2 g) dried thyme

1 cup (140 g) frozen peas

METHOD

Preheat the oven to 400°F (200°C, gas mark 6, fan 180°C). In a large bowl, add the chicken, minced garlic, chicken seasoning, salt, black pepper and lemon juice and mix to combine. Set aside.

Slice the leek into ½-inch (1-cm) rounds, break them up and scatter them over the base of a large baking tray. Place the chicken thighs on top of the leeks in an even layer and nestle the lemon slices between the chicken thighs. Add the chicken stock and drizzle the melted butter over the chicken pieces. Sprinkle over the thyme leaves and bake in the oven for 30 minutes.

Carefully remove the tray from the oven and scatter over the frozen peas. Do not be tempted to flip the chicken thighs—we want them to crisp up! Pop the tray back into to oven and cook for 15 minutes, or until the chicken thighs are cooked through and the skin is golden and crispy. Serve with sides of choice (see recipe introduction for suggestions) and spoon the remaining lemony flavored juices over the chicken pieces.

STORAGE & REHEATING

Store leftovers in the refrigerator for up to 3 days or freeze for up to 3 months. Thaw the chicken if frozen, and reheat it in a baking dish in the oven at 400°F (200°C, gas mark 6, fan 180°C) for 15 to 20 minutes, or until completely warmed through. Alternatively, you can reheat it in the microwave on the high setting in 1-minute intervals until the chicken is completely warmed through.

MAKE-AHEAD

FREEZER FRIENDLY

ALLERGEN: DAIRY

SOURCE OF IRON & PROTEIN

Serves:
Makes 8 to 10 fritters

Prep Time:
8 minutes

Cook Time:
6 to 8 minutes per batch

READY IN 30 MINUTES OR LESS

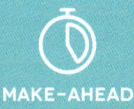

MAKE-AHEAD

FREEZER FRIENDLY

LUNCHBOX FRIENDLY

VEGETARIAN

ALLERGEN: EGGS

Crispy Sweet Corn Fritters

If you are like me and you always seem to have a can of sweet corn hanging out in the pantry, then you will appreciate having this simple yet flavorful recipe on hand! The subtly sweet, golden and crisp fritters are simple to make and perfect for quick lunches or snacks. Unlike typical corn fritters, I prefer to blend the corn kernels right into the batter, as it brings out the sweetness of the sweet corn and gives the fritters a fluffier texture. I recommend serving these fritters with my Homemade Marinara Dipping Sauce (page 127) or a generous helping of guacamole.

INGREDIENTS

2 (7-oz [200-g]) cans sweet corn, drained and rinsed

2 large eggs

3 scallions (white and green parts), roughly chopped

1 cup (125 g) all-purpose flour

½ tsp baking powder

½ tsp garlic granules or powder

Salt and black pepper, to taste

2 tbsp (30 ml) avocado oil or high-heat oil of choice, for shallow frying

METHOD

Add the sweet corn, eggs, chopped scallions, flour, baking powder, garlic granules, salt and black pepper into a blender and blend on high speed for 1 to 2 minutes, or until you have a well-formed batter. It will be lumpy, which is fine.

Heat a large nonstick frying pan over medium heat and add the avocado oil. Once the oil is hot, spoon ¼ cup (60 ml) of the batter to the frying pan. Fry the fritters for 3 to 4 minutes on each side, or until the fritters are golden and the corners become crisp. Transfer the fritters to a layer of paper towels to drain. Allow to cool sufficiently before serving.

STORAGE & REHEATING

Store the fritters in an airtight container in the refrigerator for up to 3 days. To freeze, stack the fritters between sheets of parchment paper in a freezer bag and freeze them for up to 3 months. Thaw the fritters in the refrigerator or at room temperature before reheating uncovered in the oven at 350°F (180°C, gas mark 4, fan 160°C) for about 10 to 15 minutes, or until warmed through.

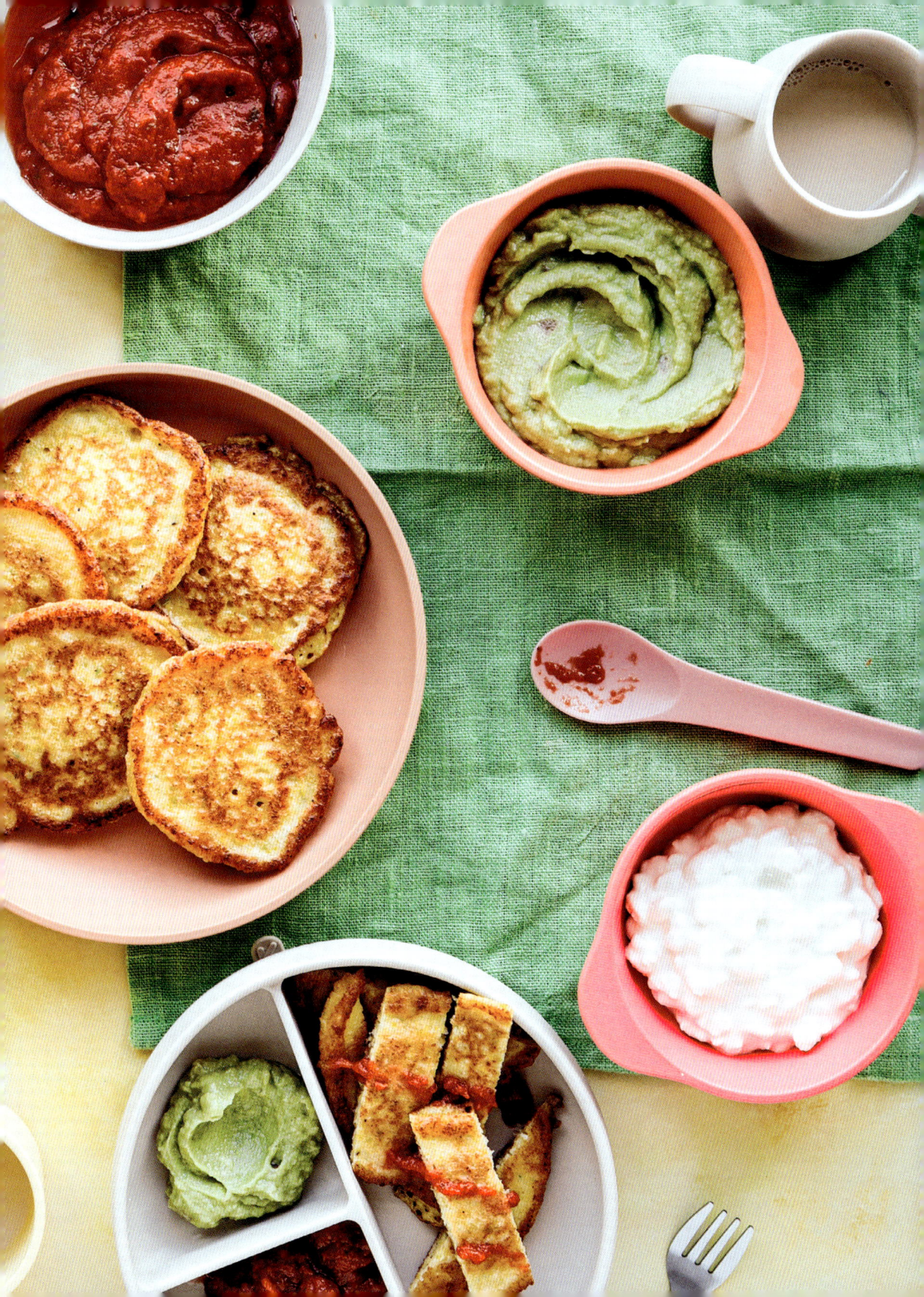

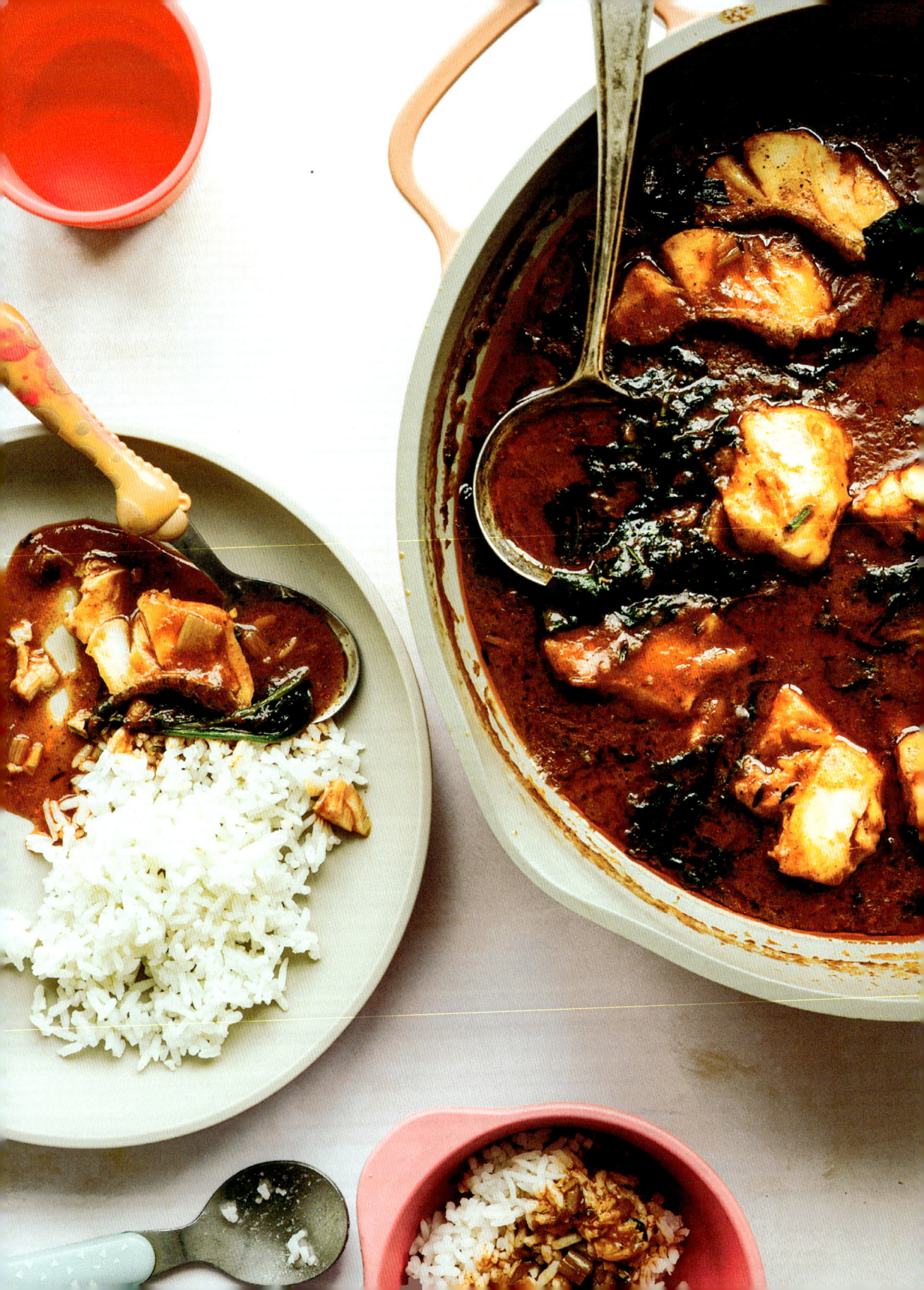

Spinach & Cod Mild Coconut Curry

I couldn't create another cookbook without including a curry recipe that can be enjoyed by the whole family! We love all types of curries from all over the world, and one of my favorite quick offerings is this super simple Jamaican-inspired curry that comes together in less than 30 minutes. I like using cod here because it's a light and unintimidating white fish that kids tend to enjoy, and it cooks very quickly, but you can also use shrimp if you prefer. Mild curry powder is the star of the show here, offering a big flavor payoff but without the heat—and it complements the cod beautifully, aromatically infusing the delicate fish without being overpowering, and bounces off the mellow notes of the coconut milk. I serve this curry with fluffy white basmati rice, but you can serve it with any grain you prefer.

Serves: 4

Prep Time: 5 minutes

Cook Time: 16 to 18 minutes

INGREDIENTS

2 tbsp (30 ml) avocado or olive oil, for frying

4 scallions, finely chopped

2 garlic cloves, minced

2 tsp (4 g) mild curry powder

½ tsp ground ginger

2 tsp fresh thyme leaves or 1 tsp dried thyme

1 tbsp (15 g) tomato paste

1 (14-oz [420-ml]) can full-fat coconut milk

¾ cup (180 ml) chicken stock

12.5 oz (350 g) skinless, boneless fresh cod, cut into 2-inch (5-cm) chunks

2 cups (60 g) tightly packed fresh baby spinach

Salt and black pepper, to taste

METHOD

Heat a large, wide-based pan over medium heat and add the avocado oil. Once the oil is hot, add the chopped scallions, minced garlic, curry powder, ground ginger and thyme. Mix to combine and cook for 2 minutes, stirring often.

Add the tomato paste, coconut milk and chicken stock and mix until well combined and the tomato paste has melted into the liquid. Bring to a boil, then turn the heat down to medium-low and simmer for 5 to 6 minutes, or until the curry sauce starts to thicken. The curry will look pale to start, but the color will deepen as it cooks down.

Add the cod in an even layer, nestling the pieces in the sauce but not submerging them. Turn the heat down to low, cover with a lid and cook for 8 to 10 minutes, or until the cod is flaky and cooked through. Remove the lid and scatter the baby spinach over the top of the curry. Cover and cook for 2 minutes, or until the spinach starts to wilt. Add some salt and black pepper and gently stir the cod and baby spinach into the curry sauce, being careful not to break up the delicate fish. Allow to cool sufficiently before serving.

STORAGE & REHEATING

Leftovers can be stored in an airtight container in the refrigerator for up to 3 days. Reheat in the microwave (covered) on the high setting for 30-second intervals until warmed through.

30 READY IN 30 MINUTES OR LESS

ONE-POT MEAL

SOURCE OF PROTEIN

NUTRITIOUS & DELICIOUS MAINS THAT LITTLE ONES WILL LOVE

Serves: 6

Prep Time: 10 minutes

Cook Time: 45 to 50 minutes

MAKE-AHEAD

VEGETARIAN

Chunky Veggie Pasta Bake

We all need a good pasta bake recipe on hand—they are low effort, tasty and a great crowd pleaser. What's more, pasta sauces are super easy to make at home! I have been making this rich and hearty veggie pasta bake for my family for over 6 years now, perfecting it along the way, and I finally have the perfect ratio of veggies to sauce—speaking of which, this recipe is packed with seven glorious veggies! I like to leave the veggies chunky in the sauce, as they add great texture, but feel free to puree the sauce before adding it to the pasta if you have a picky toddler who is still learning to enjoy bigger pieces of vegetables. I often make the sauce ahead of time and freeze it; it intensifies in flavor and makes this the quickest and easiest weeknight meal.

INGREDIENTS

17.5 oz (500 g) penne pasta

2 tbsp (30 ml) avocado or olive oil, for frying

1 large brown onion, peeled and finely diced

1 red bell pepper, cut into chunks

2 garlic cloves, minced

1 small eggplant, diced

1 small zucchini, sliced into half moons

1 cup (70 g) button mushrooms, diced

1 cup (110 g) shredded carrot

1 cup (150 g) cherry or grape tomatoes, halved

2 tsp (4 g) dried mixed herbs

Salt and black pepper, to taste

2 (15-oz [400-g]) jars passata or sieved tomatoes

1 tbsp (15 g) tomato paste

2 tbsp (30 ml) Worcestershire sauce

1 cup (115 g) grated cheese or nondairy cheese of choice

METHOD

Bring a large pot of water to a boil over high heat. Add the pasta and cook it according to the package instructions. Drain 5 minutes before the suggested cooking time and set aside.

Meanwhile, preheat the oven to 400°F (200°C, gas mark 6, fan 180°C) and heat a large, wide-based pan over medium heat and add the avocado oil. Once the oil is hot, add the diced onion and diced red bell pepper and cook for 2 to 3 minutes, stirring often. Add the garlic, mix and cook for 1 minute.

Add the diced eggplant, sliced zucchini, diced mushroom and shredded carrot and mix to combine. Cook for 3 to 4 to minutes, or until the veggies start to soften. Add the halved cherry tomatoes, mixed herbs, salt and black pepper, and mix to combine. Cook for 2 minutes, stirring often.

Add the passata, tomato paste and Worcestershire sauce, mix thoroughly and bring to a boil. Turn the heat down to low and cover with a lid. Simmer for 5 minutes.

Add the cooked pasta to the pot and mix until all of the pasta is coated. Transfer to a large baking dish and sprinkle over the grated cheese. Cook in the oven for 25 to 30 minutes, or until the cheese is golden and bubbling. Allow to cool sufficiently before serving.

STORAGE & REHEATING

Leftovers can be stored in the refrigerator for up to 3 days. To reheat, place the pasta bake in the oven (covered) at 350°F (180°C, gas mark 4, fan 160°C) for 15 to 20 minutes, or until fully heated through.

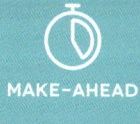

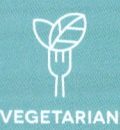

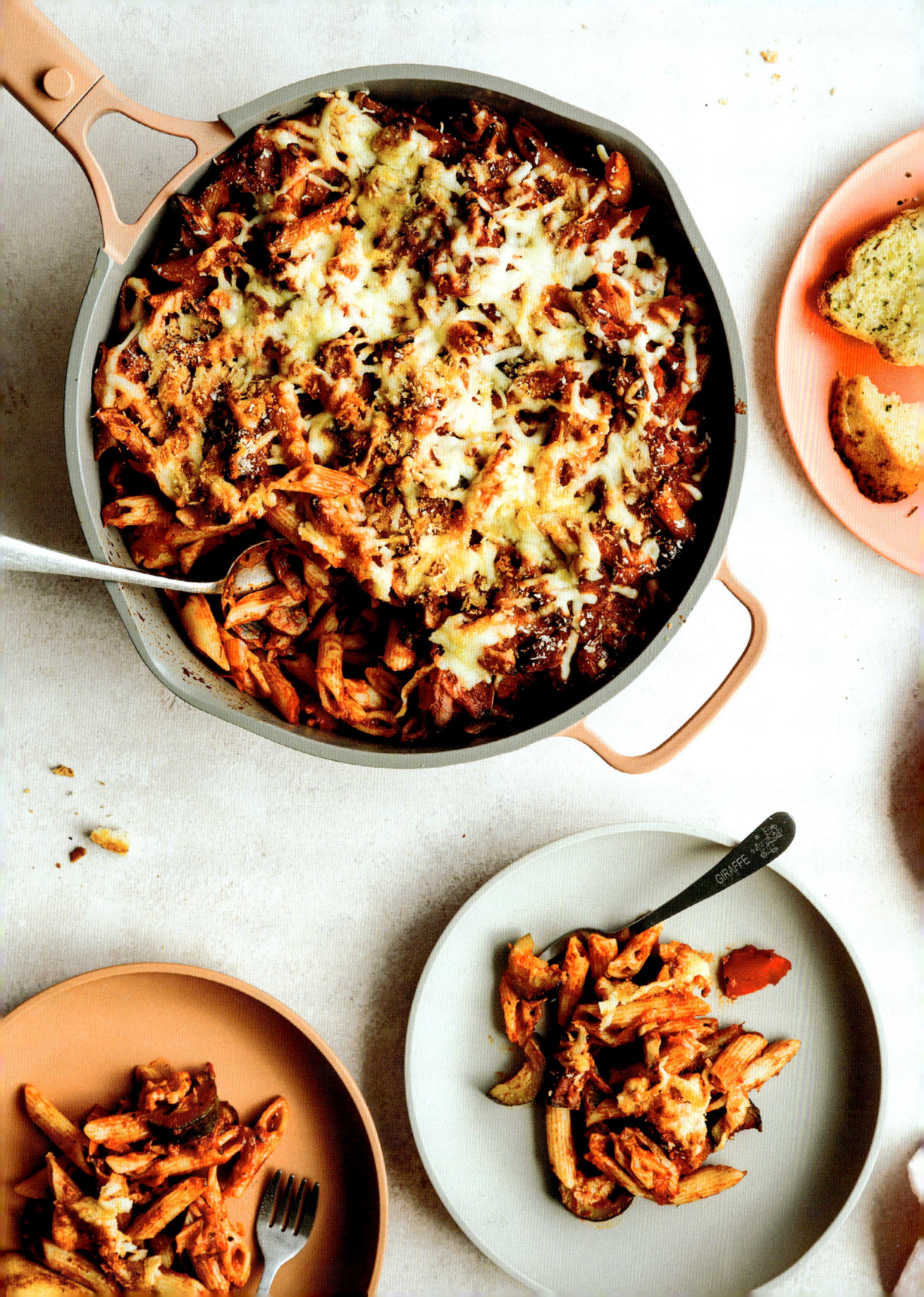

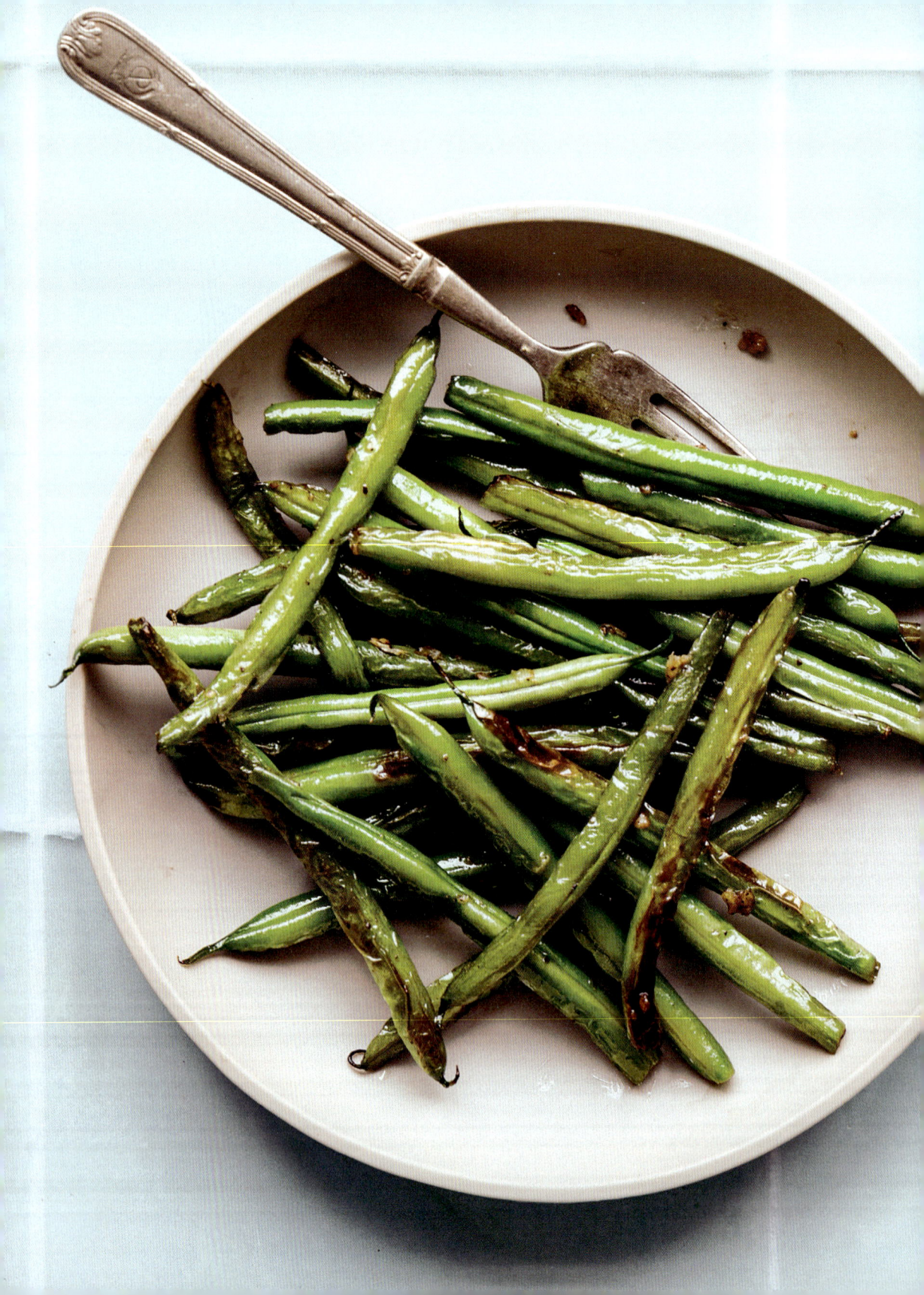

CHAPTER 5

Something Different on the Side

One thing about side dishes is that even though they can make or break a meal, we often pay them the least attention because we simply don't have the time or energy to think up something new or exciting. In this chapter, you will find a selection of simple side dishes that will help to keep things interesting and varied at mealtimes, including some exciting ways to pump up veggies and make them more appealing to toddlers!

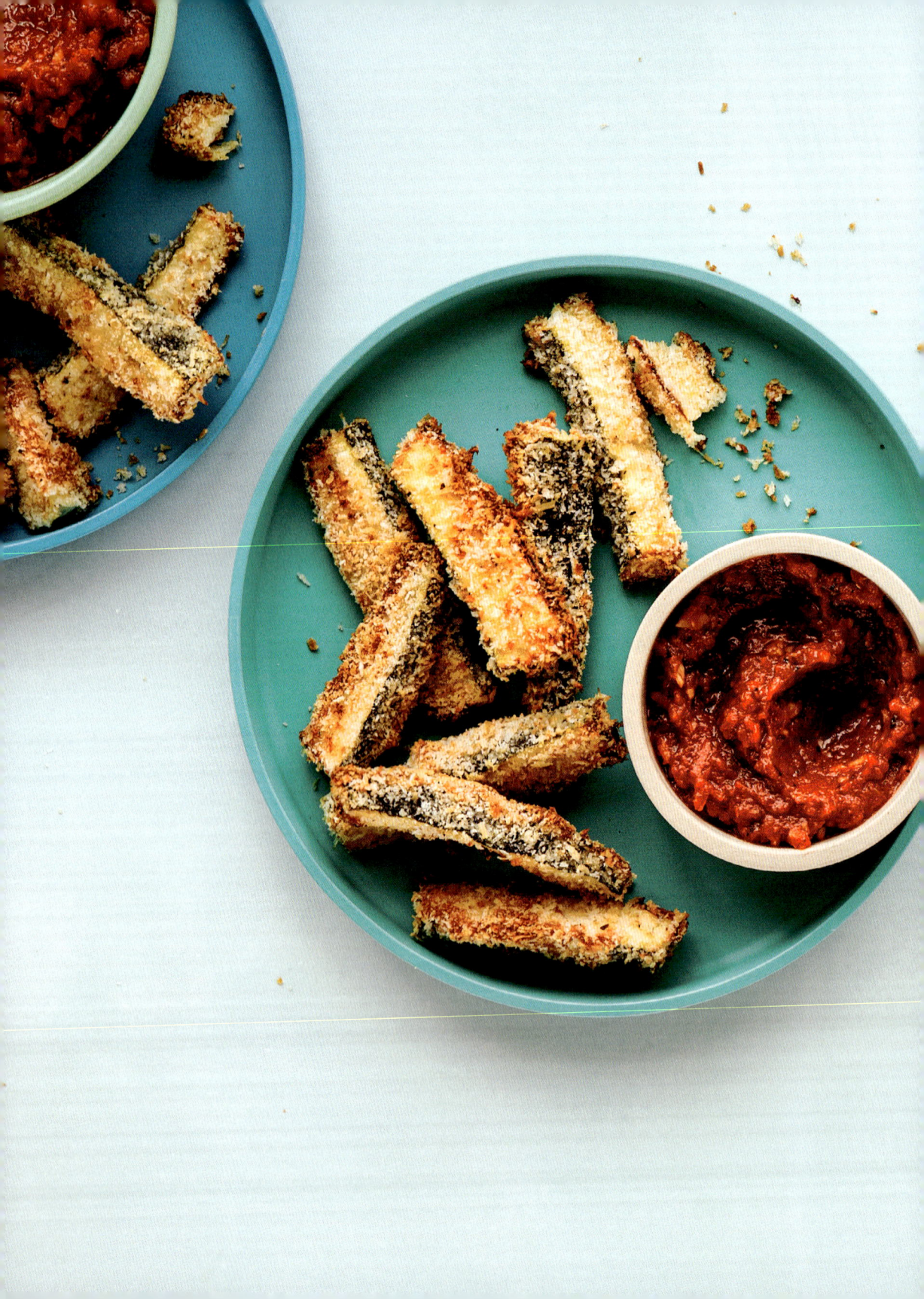

Crispy Zucchini Fries

Zucchini is often an unpopular vegetable with kids, which I suspect could be because of the texture. It's so easy to overcook and it can quickly turn into mush, which is not the most appealing texture for a vegetable. My go-to solution for this is to cut this green vegetable into sticks, roll it in a flavorful crumb and bake it in the oven until it's beautifully crisp and golden on the outside, which complements its soft, buttery texture on the inside—my kids think they are the best thing ever and they pair brilliantly with my Homemade Marinara Dipping Sauce (page 127). The almond meal not only provides a boost of iron, protein and healthy fats, but it also helps the crumb to adhere to the zucchini and not slide off. If your child has an almond allergy, you can substitute with more panko breadcrumbs, but be sure to handle the sticks with care.

Serves: 4

Prep Time: 10 minutes

Cook Time: 18 to 22 minutes

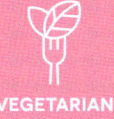

INGREDIENTS

- ¼ cup (25 g) almond meal (see notes)
- ½ cup (30 g) panko breadcrumbs
- ¼ cup (25 g) grated parmesan cheese or 2 tbsp (20 g) nutritional yeast (nondairy option)
- ½ tsp garlic granules or powder
- ½ tsp onion granules or powder
- Salt and black pepper, to taste
- 2 large eggs, lightly beaten
- 2 medium zucchinis, cut into ½-inch (1-cm) stick shapes
- Nonstick cooking spray, as needed

METHOD

Preheat the oven to 425°F (220°C, gas mark 7, fan 200°C) and line a large baking sheet with parchment paper.

In a large, wide and shallow bowl, add the almond meal, panko breadcrumbs, parmesan cheese, garlic granules, onion granules, salt and black pepper, and mix until well combined. In a separate bowl, whisk the eggs until lightly foamy.

Place the zucchini sticks into the bowl with the whisked eggs and mix until they are all coated evenly. Using cooking tongs, take a zucchini stick and roll it in the breadcrumb mixture until all sides are coated, lightly pressing on each stick to help the breadcrumb mixture adhere to the sticks.

Arrange the zucchini on the lined baking sheet, making sure they are not touching. Spray generously with the nonstick cooking spray and bake in the oven for 18 to 22 minutes, or until crisp and golden. Allow to cool sufficiently before serving.

STORAGE & REHEATING

Leftovers can be stored in an airtight container in the refrigerator for up to 2 days. To reheat, place the zucchini fries on a lined baking sheet and respray with some nonstick cooking spray. Reheat in the oven at 375°F (190°C, gas mark 5, fan 170°C) for 8 to 10 minutes, or until crisp and warmed through.

NOTES

Almond meal is also known as ground almonds and is typically found in the baking section at the grocery store.

VEGETARIAN

ALLERGEN: EGGS

SOURCE OF HEALTHY FATS, IRON & PROTEIN

SOMETHING DIFFERENT ON THE SIDE

Serves:
Makes 4 slices

Prep Time:
4 minutes

Cook Time:
16 minutes

Cheesy Garlic Bread

Good old bread and cheese has long been a comforting combo that my kids will reliably eat, so I'm always looking for ways to keep these on rotation while also keeping them interesting. Although simplistic in its production, this recipe does not lack in flavor and has proven to be popular with both the kids and the adults in my family. I like to pair it with my super quick 20-Minute Iron-Rich Tomato Soup (page 59), but it can also be served as an easy filling lunch with a fruit or veggie on the side.

INGREDIENTS

4 slices sourdough bread, or bread of choice

¼ cup (60 g) unsalted butter or nondairy butter of choice

2 cloves garlic minced (or more or less to taste)

1 cup (115 g) grated mozzarella or nondairy cheese of choice

2 tsp (1 g) finely chopped fresh parsley or 1 tsp dried parsley

METHOD

Preheat the oven to 400°F (200°C, gas mark 6, fan 180°C) and line a baking sheet with parchment paper. Arrange the bread on the baking sheet.

In a small microwave-safe bowl, add the butter and the minced garlic. Microwave on high for 30 seconds, or until the butter has melted. Ensure the butter and garlic are thoroughly mixed together, then use a pastry brush to evenly distribute half of the mixture over the bread slices. Bake in the oven for 6 minutes.

Carefully remove the baking sheet from the oven and turn the bread slices over. Brush the rest of the garlic butter mixture over the bread slices and top each slice with the grated mozzarella. Sprinkle each slice evenly with the chopped fresh parsley. Bake in the oven for around 10 minutes, or until the cheese is melted, golden and bubbly. Best served freshly cooked.

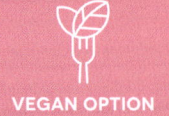

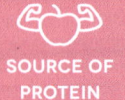

30 READY IN 30 MINUTES OR LESS

VEGAN OPTION

SOURCE OF PROTEIN

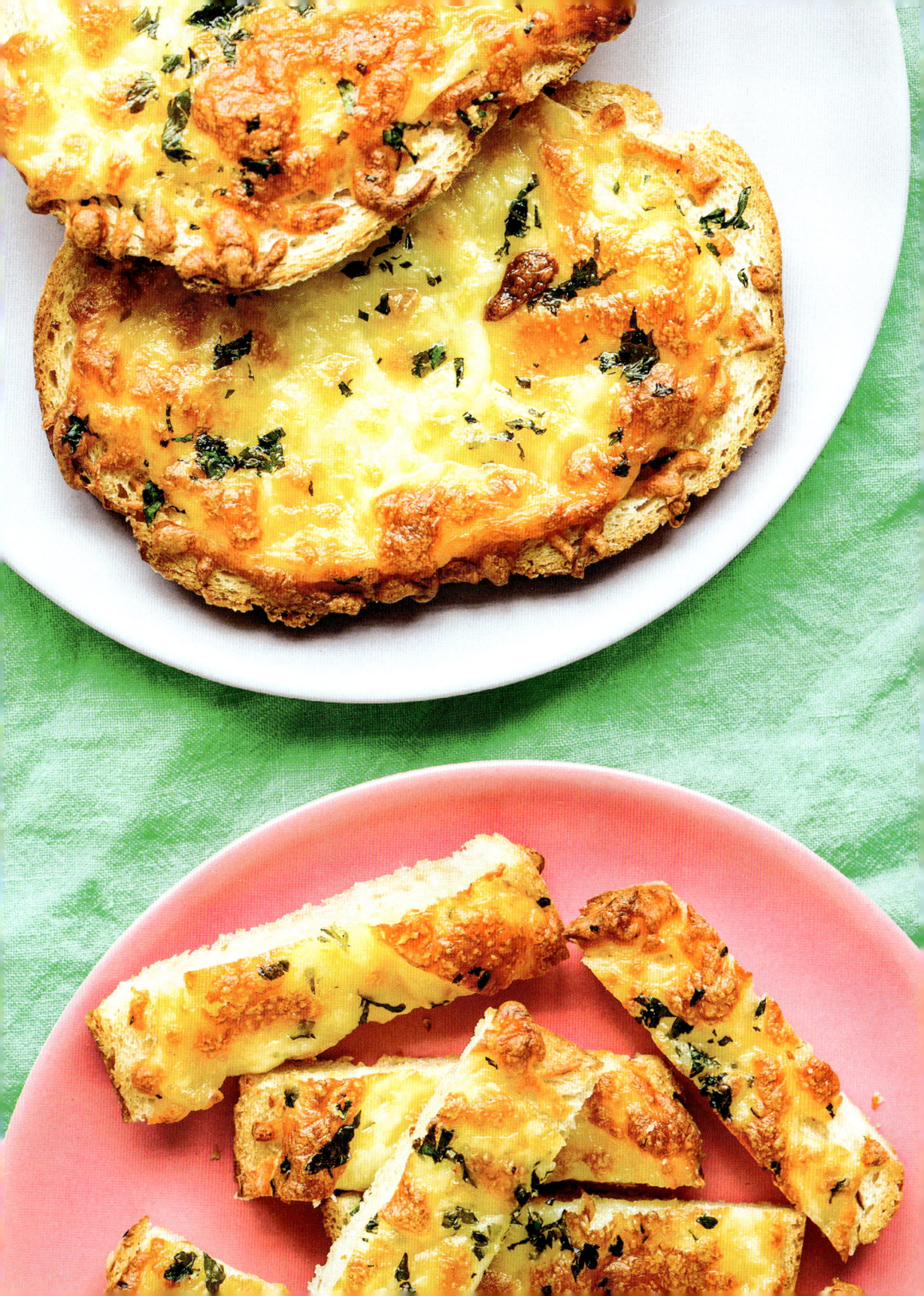

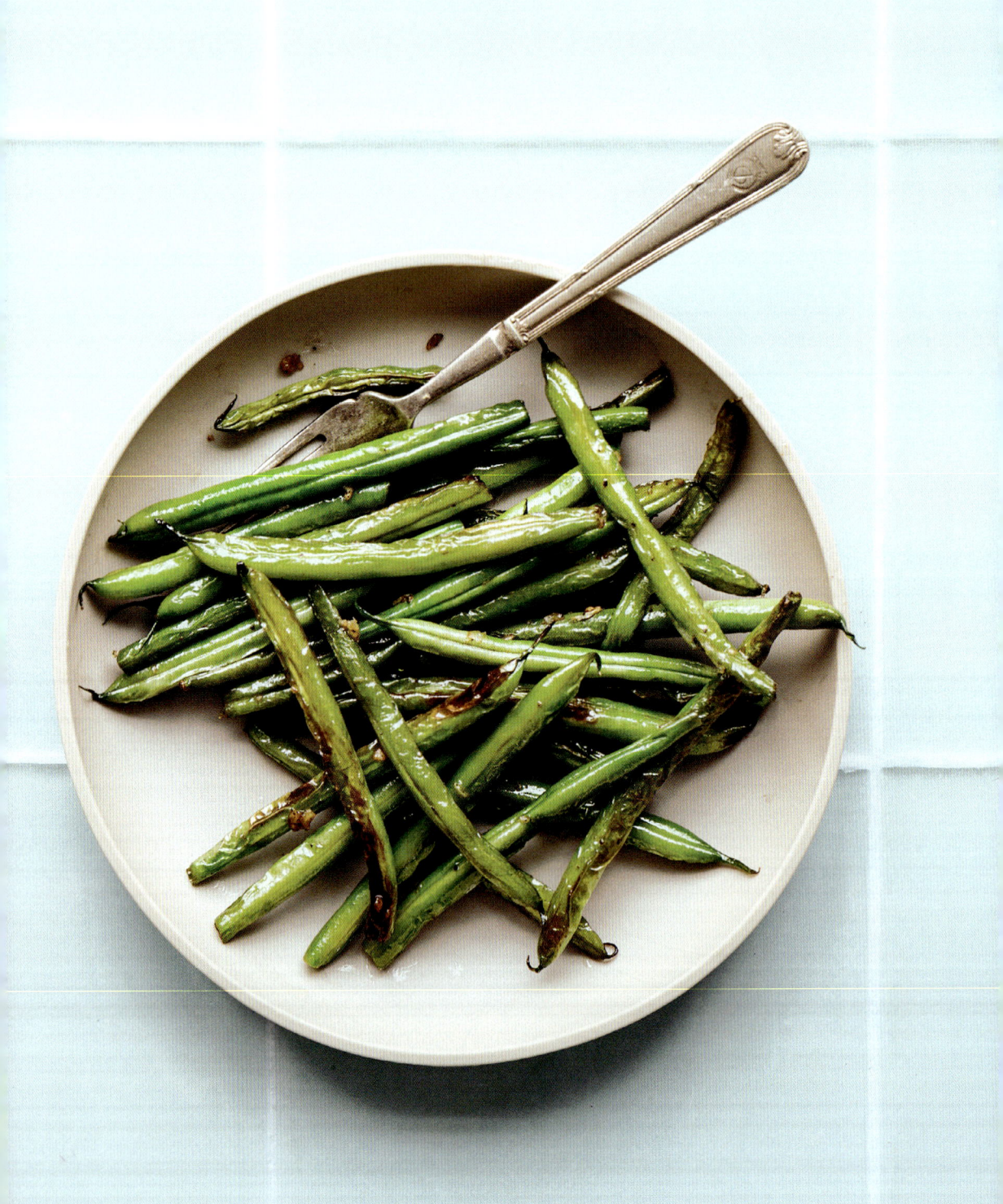

Sautéed Green Beans

Green beans are a staple in many a household and for good reason—they are widely available, affordable and incredibly nutritious! They are most definitely on heavy rotation in my house, which is why I like to switch things up to keep my kids from getting bored. In this recipe, the green beans do a great job of soaking up the warming flavors from the butter and garlic, and cooking them covered allows them to steam through and become incredibly tender without overly crisping up or burning their skin. A sure winner at any table!

Serves: 4

Prep Time: 5 minutes

Cook Time: 15 minutes

INGREDIENTS

2 tbsp (30 ml) avocado or olive oil

1 tbsp (15 ml) unsalted butter or nondairy butter of choice

14oz (400 g) green beans, woody ends trimmed

Salt and black pepper, to taste

2 garlic cloves, minced

METHOD

Heat a large nonstick frying pan over medium heat and add the avocado oil and butter. Once the oil is hot and the butter has melted, add the green beans, salt and black pepper and toss them in the pan, making sure they are evenly coated in the oil and butter. Cover with a lid, turn the heat down to medium-low and cook for 10 minutes, stirring halfway through.

Add the minced garlic and toss until well combined. Cover with a lid and cook for 5 minutes, or until fork tender. Serve warm.

STORAGE & REHEATING

Store in an airtight container in the refrigerator for up to 3 days. To reheat, place the green beans in a baking dish, cover and pop them in the oven at 350°F (180°C, gas mark 4, fan 160°C) for around 7 to 8 minutes, or until heated through. Alternatively, you can reheat them in the microwave (covered) on the high setting for 30-second intervals until heated through.

30 READY IN UNDER 30 MINUTES

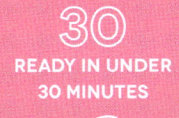

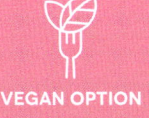

VEGAN OPTION

Serves:
4

Prep Time:
4 minutes

Cook Time:
15 minutes

Easy Garlic Noodles

This is probably the easiest recipe in this cookbook, but it is by no means lacking! I love to jazz up pasta with my super easy garlic-infused oil—it's a great flavor boost for adults, but also a great option if you have a picky toddler that refuses to have any sauces on their pasta. You can introduce them to new flavors on their pasta in a low-pressure way, not to mention that they get that extra boost of healthy fats, which is essential for their growing bodies and brains. Feel free to skip the parsley if your little one is not keen on anything green—you can gradually incorporate this over time, if you wish.

INGREDIENTS

14 oz (400g) spaghetti or linguine

3 tbsp (45 ml) olive oil

2 garlic cloves, minced, or more or less to taste

2 tbsp (6 g) finely chopped fresh parsley (optional)

Salt and black pepper, to taste

METHOD

Bring a large pot of water to a boil over high heat. Once the water comes to a rolling boil, add the spaghetti and cook it according to the package instructions.

Five minutes before the pasta is cooked, heat a large, nonstick, wide-based pan over medium heat and add the olive oil. Once the oil is hot, add the minced garlic and cook for 1 minute, or until fragrant, stirring often.

Drain the cooked pasta thoroughly and add it straight to the pan of garlic-infused oil along with the chopped fresh parsley (if using) and some salt and black pepper. Toss the spaghetti until everything is coated in the oil. Serve immediately.

STORAGE

Leftovers can be stored in an airtight container in the refrigerator for up to 2 days.

30 — READY IN 30 MINUTES OR LESS

VEGAN

SOURCE OF HEALTHY FATS

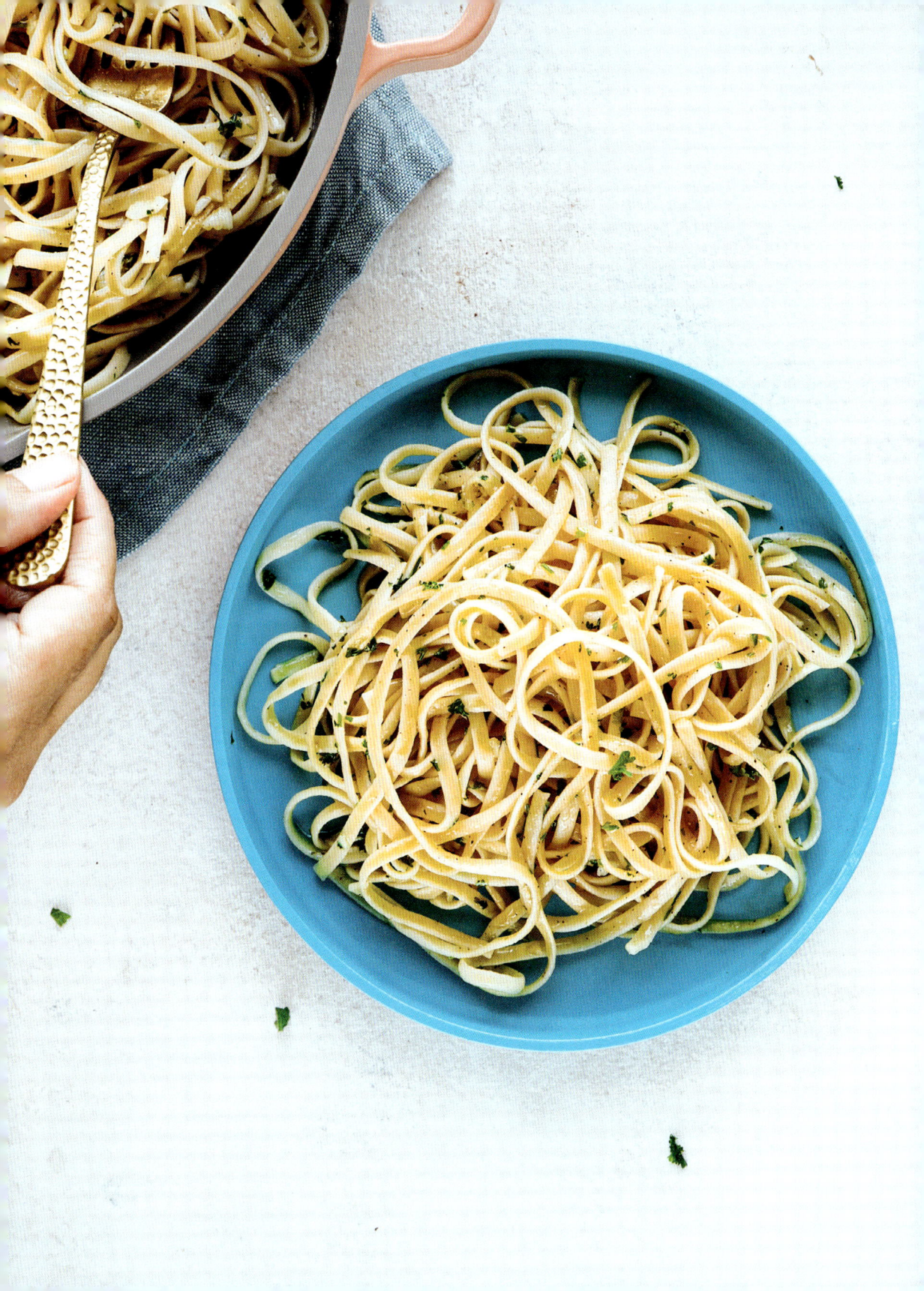

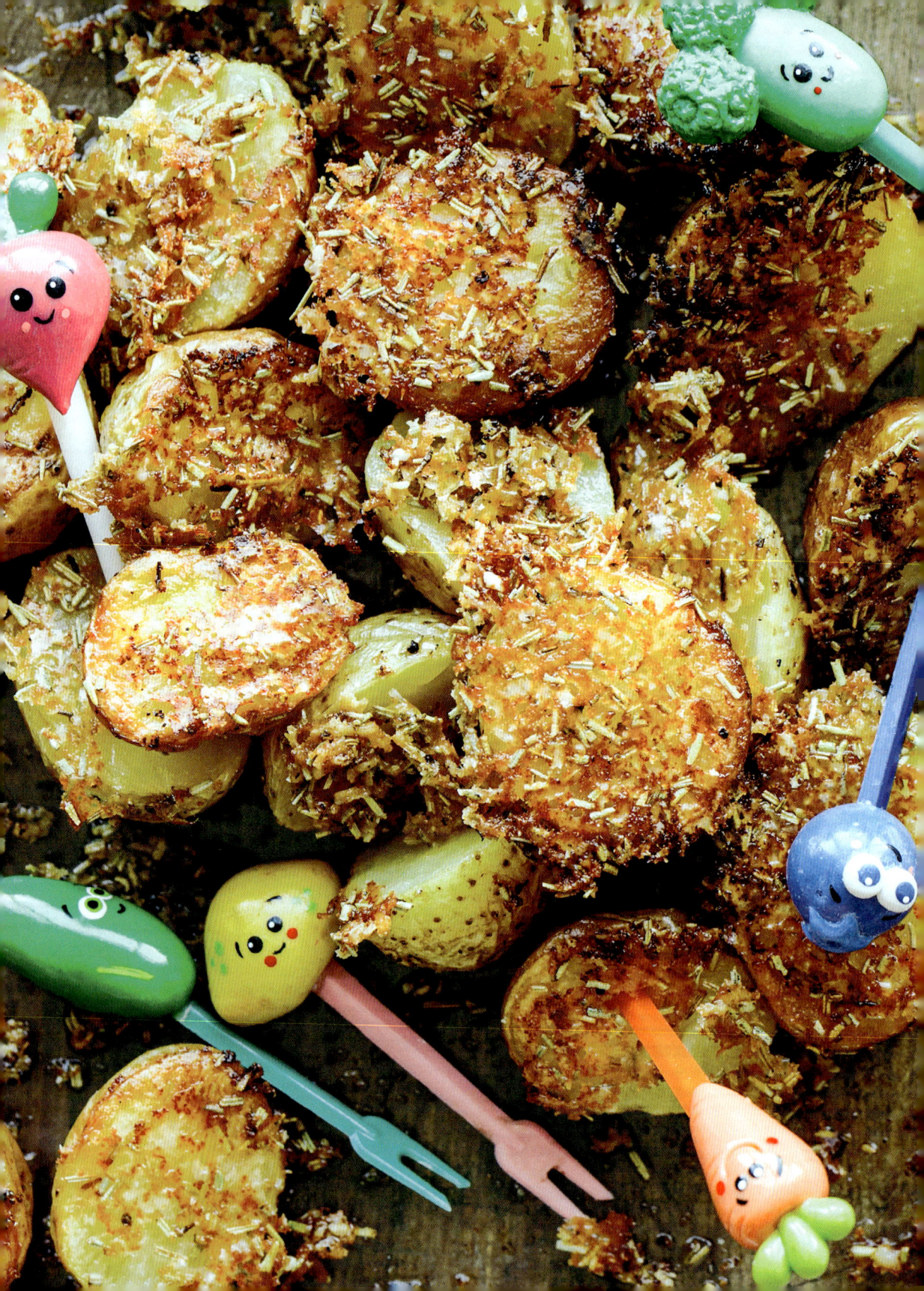

Parmesan Crusted Roasties

I like to think of these dangerously addictive parmesan-crusted roasted potatoes as a cheat version of regular roasties, but with even more flavor, and they pair well with many recipes in this book. The most work you will do here is grate some parmesan, halve the potatoes and mix the crust. After that, everything is dumped into a baking tray and left to its own devices in the oven—what's more, since kids tend to adore potatoes and cheese, this side dish will be received with joy! I prefer to use freshly grated parmesan for maximum crispiness, but feel free to use the finer, sandier type if preferred—just ensure you stick with fresh parmesan and not dried, because the dried variety burns very easily and becomes bitter.

Serves: 6

Prep Time: 8 minutes

Cook Time: 35 to 40 minutes

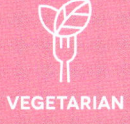

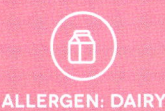

INGREDIENTS

½ cup (50 g) finely grated parmesan cheese

½ tsp garlic granules or powder

½ tsp onion granules or powder

1 tsp dried rosemary

3 tbsp (45 ml) avocado or olive oil, divided

1 lb (500 g) baby potatoes, halved lengthwise

Salt and black pepper, to taste

METHOD

Preheat the oven to 400°F (200°C, gas mark 6, fan 180°C).

In a small bowl, combine the grated parmesan, garlic granules, onion granules and dried rosemary. Set aside.

In a large baking sheet, drizzle over 1 tablespoon (15 ml) of avocado oil and use a pastry brush to spread it evenly over the surface of the tray.

Sprinkle the parmesan mixture evenly over the oil on the baking tray, making sure all of the surface is coated. Place the baby potatoes cut side down over the parmesan mixture, pressing down firmly on each potato so it adheres to the mixture. Drizzle the remaining 2 tablespoons (30 ml) of oil evenly over the potatoes and season with salt and black pepper.

Bake in the oven for 35 to 40 minutes, or until the potatoes are fork tender and golden in color. Remove the tray from the oven and rest the potatoes for 2 minutes. Using a butter knife or small spatula, gently flip each potato over, being careful not to detach the parmesan crust. Allow to cool sufficiently before serving.

STORAGE & REHEATING

Leftovers can be stored in the refrigerator for up to 3 days. Reheat them in the oven at 350°F (180°C, gas mark 4, fan 160°C) for 10 to 15 minutes, or until they are warmed through and crisp.

VEGETARIAN

ALLERGEN: DAIRY

SOURCE OF FIBER

SOMETHING DIFFERENT ON THE SIDE

Serves:
Makes 1½ cups (360 g)

Prep Time:
5 minutes + 15 minutes chill time

Lemon Garlic Dip

Dips are often popular with toddlers, and they can encourage even the pickiest of eaters to at least interact with foods they are still learning to like—licking dip off broccoli still counts as a positive food exposure, even if they don't eat the broccoli! I love this dip because of its versatility—it pairs well with cooked foods, such as fritters or fries, as well as raw veggies. The rich punchy flavors appeal to both adults and kids, and you can adjust the flavor intensity to suit your family's taste buds.

INGREDIENTS

1 cup (240 ml) mayonnaise or plant-based mayonnaise of choice

½ cup (140 g) full-fat plain Greek or natural yogurt or nondairy plain yogurt of choice

½ garlic clove, minced, or more or less to taste (see notes)

2 tbsp (30 ml) freshly squeezed lemon juice

1 tbsp (3 g) chopped fresh dill or 1 tsp dried dill

Salt and black pepper, to taste

METHOD
Add all of the ingredients to a medium-sized bowl and mix until well combined. Chill in the refrigerator for at least 15 minutes before serving.

STORAGE
Store in an airtight container in the refrigerator for up to a week.

NOTES
If your toddler is still learning to like the flavor of raw garlic, you can switch it out for garlic granules or powder. Start with ½ teaspoon and see how they get on, increasing the amount if desired.

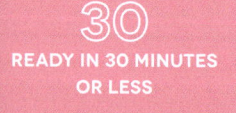

READY IN 30 MINUTES OR LESS

MAKE-AHEAD

VEGAN OPTION

SOURCE OF PROTEIN

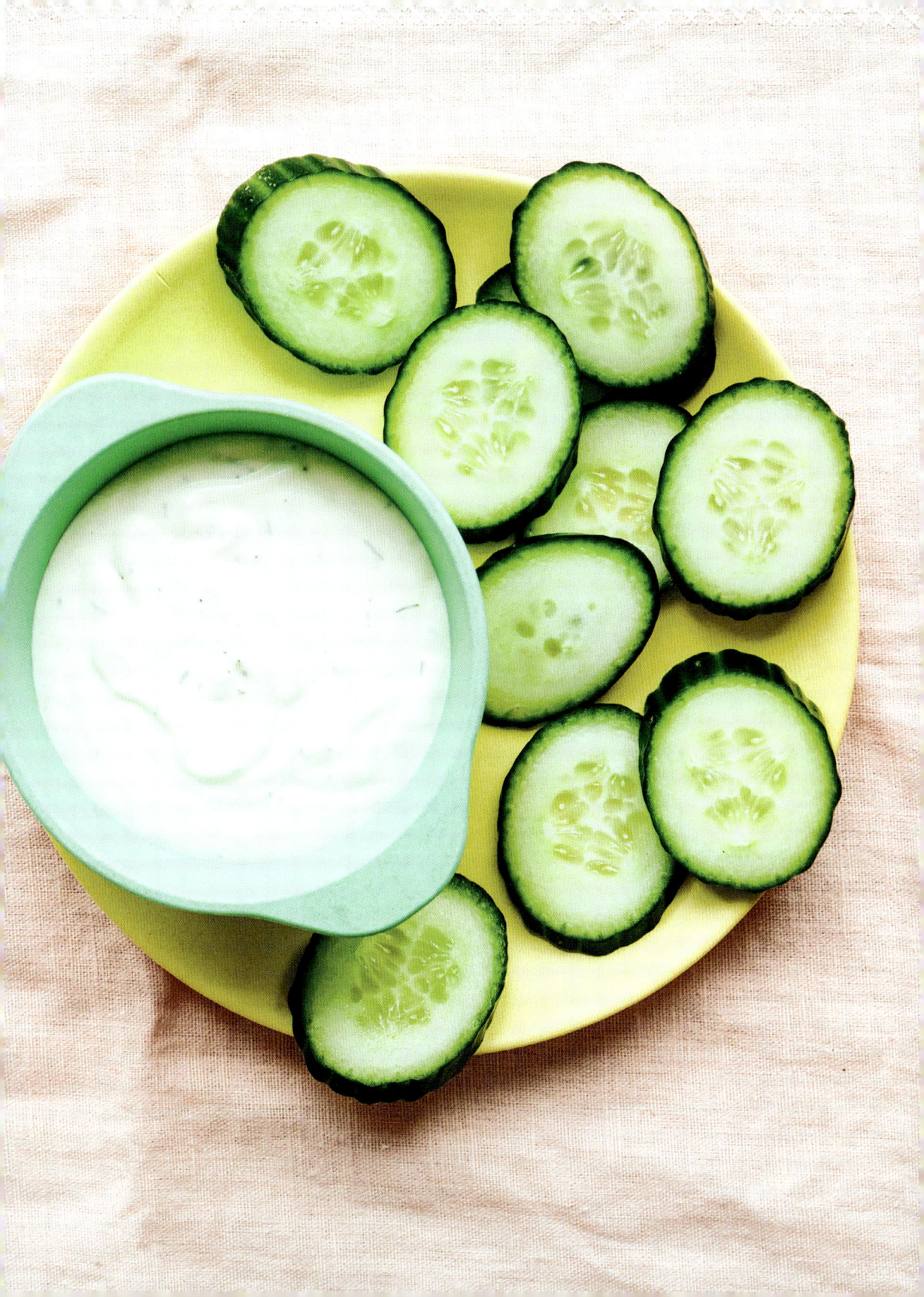

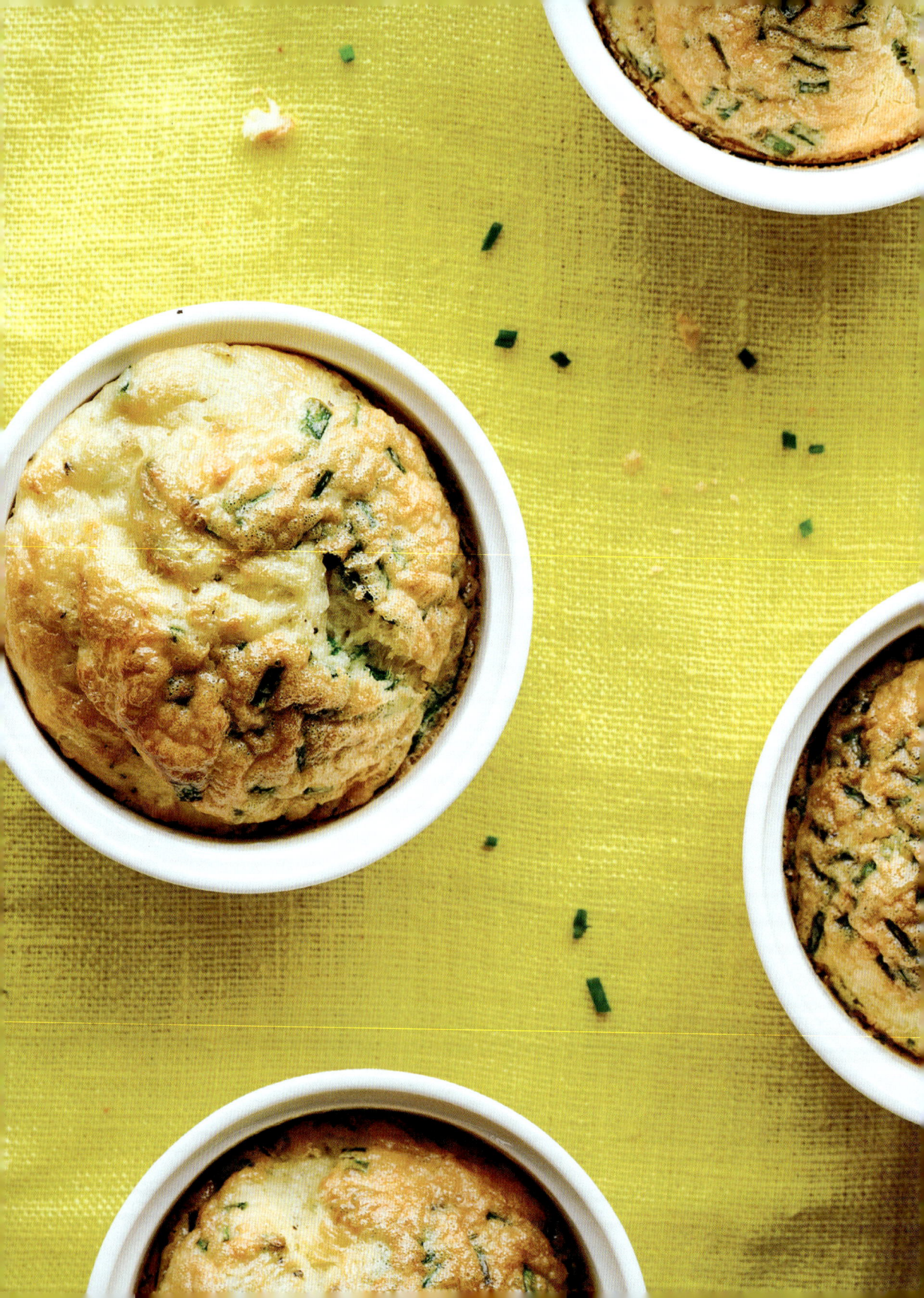

Eggy Bread Rolls

Like a cross between an egg muffin and a bread roll, this recipe makes for the perfect quick and easy side dish using the simplest of ingredients. And what's more, there is very little work required—just a bit of mixing and pouring! These rolls are light yet filling, and they're packed with iron and protein. You can flavor them in any way you like, adding herbs, spices and even some cheese if you fancy. If you don't have any ramekins, feel free to cook these in a standard-size muffin pan and shave a couple of minutes off the cooking time. I like to serve them with a slathering of butter, and they pair perfectly with my Quick-Cook Sausage & Pepper Stew (page 93).

INGREDIENTS

Nonstick cooking spray, as needed

4 large eggs

4 tsp (20 ml) melted unsalted butter

4 tsp (4 g) chopped fresh chives or 2 tsp (3 g) dried chives (optional)

¼ cup (30 g) all-purpose flour

1 tsp baking powder

Salt and black pepper, to taste

METHOD

Preheat the oven to 350°F (180°C, gas mark 4, fan 160°C) and generously spray four ramekins with nonstick cooking spray.

Add the eggs, butter, chopped chives, flour, baking powder, salt and pepper to a medium bowl and whisk until smooth. Evenly distribute the mixture between the ramekins and bake in the oven for 15 to 20 minutes, or until bouncy to the touch. Allow to cool slightly before turning out and serving.

STORAGE & REHEATING

Leftovers can be stored in an airtight container in the refrigerator for up to 3 days. Reheat in the microwave on the high setting for 30-second intervals until warmed through.

Serves: Makes 4 rolls

Prep Time: 5 minutes

Cook Time: 15 to 20 minutes

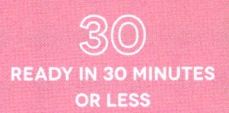

30 — READY IN 30 MINUTES OR LESS

LUNCHBOX FRIENDLY

VEGETARIAN

ALLERGEN: DAIRY & EGGS

SOURCE OF IRON & PROTEIN

Serves: 4

Prep Time: 10 minutes

Cook Time: 30 minutes

MAKE-AHEAD

VEGAN OPTION

Broccoli Mashed Potatoes

If you're looking for an interesting but easy way to incorporate more veg into your toddler's meals, then this recipe is a keeper. We call it Hulk mash in my house, and it can help to encourage kids to try broccoli if it's something they are still learning to like. You can switch out the broccoli for cooked cauliflower too, and if you wanted to add even more flavor, mixing in a sprinkling of finely grated cheese is a real crowd-pleaser. I find using a potato ricer yields the best results for a super smooth and velvety mash, but a standard potato masher works very well too. This side dish pairs excellently with my Lemony Chicken & Leek Sheet Pan (page 97)!

INGREDIENTS

2 lb (1 kg) potatoes, peeled and cut into 1-inch (2.5-cm) cubes

4 cups (350 g) broccoli florets

2/3 cup (160 ml) milk or nondairy milk of choice

1/3 cup (80 ml) butter or nondairy butter of choice

Salt and black pepper, to taste

METHOD

Bring a large pot of water to a boil over high heat and add the cubed potatoes and broccoli florets. Boil for 10 to 15 minutes, or until fork tender. Once cooked, drain the water. Alternatively, you can steam the potatoes and broccoli for 20 to 25 minutes, or until fork tender.

Meanwhile, add the milk and butter to a small microwave-safe bowl and microwave on high heat for 30 to 60 seconds, or until the butter has melted into the milk. Mix and set aside.

Using a large spoon, transfer a few pieces of the cooked potato cubes to the basket in the potato ricer and push the plunger down to force the potatoes through the holes (into a large bowl). Repeat until all of the potatoes are finished. Repeat this process with the cooked broccoli florets, adding it to the same bowl as the riced potatoes.

Once everything has been riced, add two-thirds of the milk and butter mixture, some salt and black pepper and gently mix until everything is well combined. If your mashed potato mixture isn't creamy enough, add the remaining milk and butter mixture.

If you don't have a ricer, you can mash the potatoes and broccoli together using a regular potato masher, but be sure to add the milk and butter mixture, salt and black pepper before mashing, not after.

STORAGE & REHEATING

Leftovers can be stored in an airtight container in the refrigerator for up to 2 days. To reheat, add the mashed potatoes to a pot and heat over medium heat. Add 2 tablespoons (30 ml) of milk and 1 tablespoon (15 g) of butter and mix through until the butter has melted and the potatoes are warmed through.

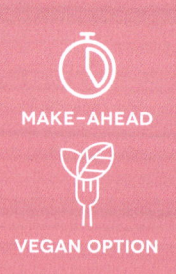

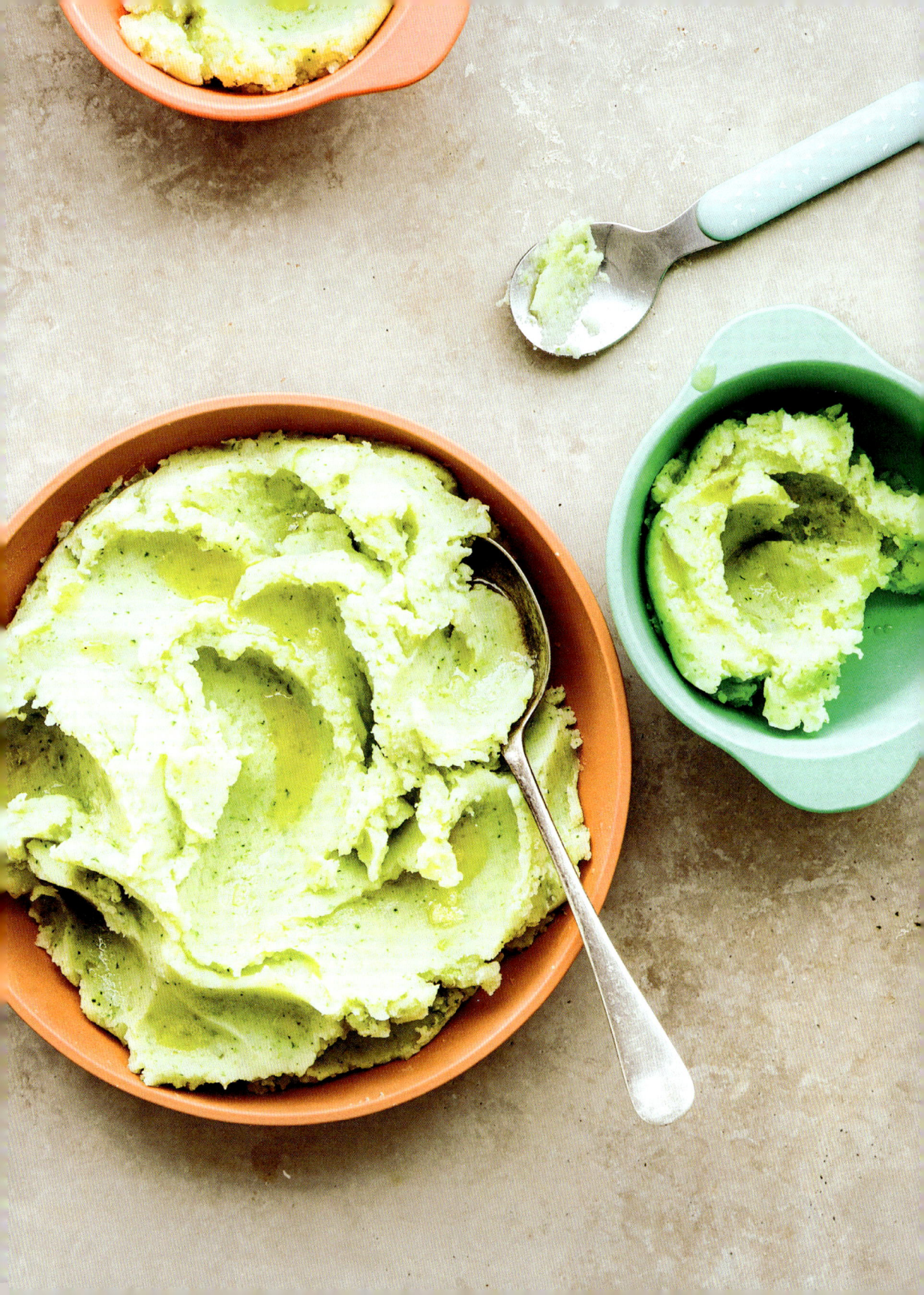

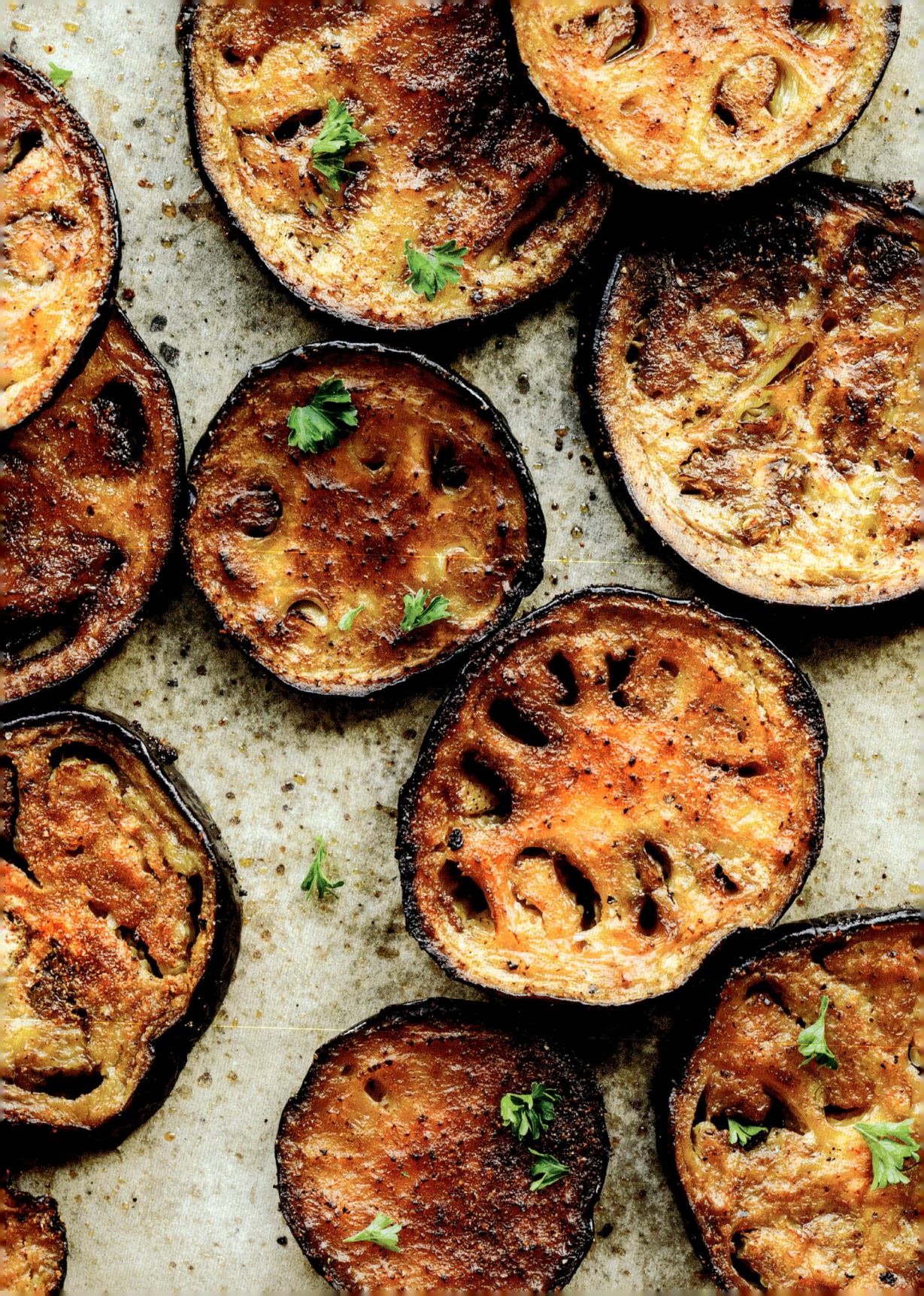

Crispy Smoky Roasted Eggplant

I have always found eggplant to be one of those vegetables that my kids either love or hate. The hate is usually reserved for the texture, as depending on how you cook it, it can be mushy or slimy. I first started testing this recipe over a year ago, and everyone in the family loved it so much, I haven't served eggplant any other way since—there's just something about the lightly smoky, salty and savory crispiness that has firmly won them over! I should add here that you shouldn't be alarmed by the amount of oil required for this recipe. Eggplant is like a sponge for oil, and the generous amount is essential for maximum crispiness, plus the avocado or olive oil makes it a great source of healthy fat for your toddler's growing body and brain!

Serves: 4

Prep Time: 6 minutes

Cook Time: 30 minutes

INGREDIENTS

1 large eggplant, washed and cut into ¾-cm (2-cm)-thick rounds

½ tsp garlic granules or powder

½ tsp onion granules or powder

½ tsp smoked paprika

Salt and black pepper, to taste

¼ cup (60 ml) avocado or olive oil, divided

METHOD

Preheat the oven to 450°F (230°C, gas mark 8, fan 210°C) and line a large baking sheet with parchment paper.

Arrange the sliced eggplant rounds on the baking sheet, making sure that they are not overlapping each other or crowding the baking sheet. Set aside.

Combine the garlic granules, onion granules, smoked paprika, salt and pepper in a small bowl and mix until combined. Sprinkle half the spice mixture evenly over the sliced eggplant rounds.

Drizzle 2 tablespoons (30 ml) of the avocado oil evenly over the sliced eggplant rounds and then turn them over. Sprinkle the remaining spice mixture over the eggplant and evenly drizzle over the remaining avocado oil.

Pop the baking sheet into the oven and cook for 15 minutes. Remove the sheet pan from the oven, turn the eggplant slices over and return to the oven to cook for a further 15 minutes, or until the eggplant slices are golden brown and crispy.

STORAGE & REHEATING

The crispy eggplant is best served right after cooking, but leftovers can be stored in an airtight container in the refrigerator for up to 2 days. Reheat uncovered in the oven at 450°F (230°C, gas mark 8, fan 210°C) for 5 to 6 minutes, or until warmed through and crispy.

VEGAN

SOURCE OF HEALTHY FATS

SOMETHING DIFFERENT ON THE SIDE

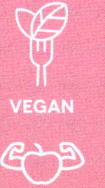

Cinnamon Roasted Sweet Potatoes

You're probably thinking that roasted sweet potatoes isn't exactly showstopping stuff, and in all honestly, you're probably right! But making a few simple changes to the spices we use and the fat we cook it in can make a big difference to the flavor payoff and take a somewhat basic side dish to another level!

Cinnamon is typically used when baking or making desserts, but this spice marries beautifully to the subtly sweet yet savory flavors of sweet potato, and the addition of the melted butter helps to create a velvety and caramelized texture that crisps up in the right places! Feel free to make these into fries if that's what your toddler prefers—I often switch between the two.

Serves: 4

Prep Time: 8 minutes

Cook Time: 30 to 35 minutes

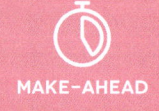

INGREDIENTS

- 2 large sweet potatoes, peeled and cut into ½-inch (1-cm) cubes
- 1 tsp ground cinnamon
- Salt and black pepper, to taste
- 3 tbsp (45 ml) melted unsalted butter or nondairy butter of choice

METHOD

Preheat the oven to 425°F (220°C, gas mark 7, fan 200°C) and line a large rimmed baking tray with parchment paper.

Place the sweet potatoes on the baking tray and add the cinnamon, salt and pepper. Use two large spoons to toss them together until all the cubes of sweet potato are coated. Arrange the sweet potato cubes in an even layer, making sure they are not touching, and drizzle the melted butter over.

Roast them in the oven for 30 to 35 minutes, or until the sweet potatoes are fork tender and golden and crispy on the edges. Do not stir or turn over the potatoes during cooking. Allow to cool sufficiently before serving.

STORAGE & REHEATING

Store in an airtight container in the refrigerator for up to 5 days or freeze for up to a month. Reheat the thawed potatoes in a baking dish (covered) in the oven at 350°F (180°C, gas mark 4, fan 160°C) for 10 minutes, or until warmed through.

MAKE-AHEAD

FREEZER FRIENDLY

VEGAN OPTION

SOURCE OF FIBER & HEALTHY FATS

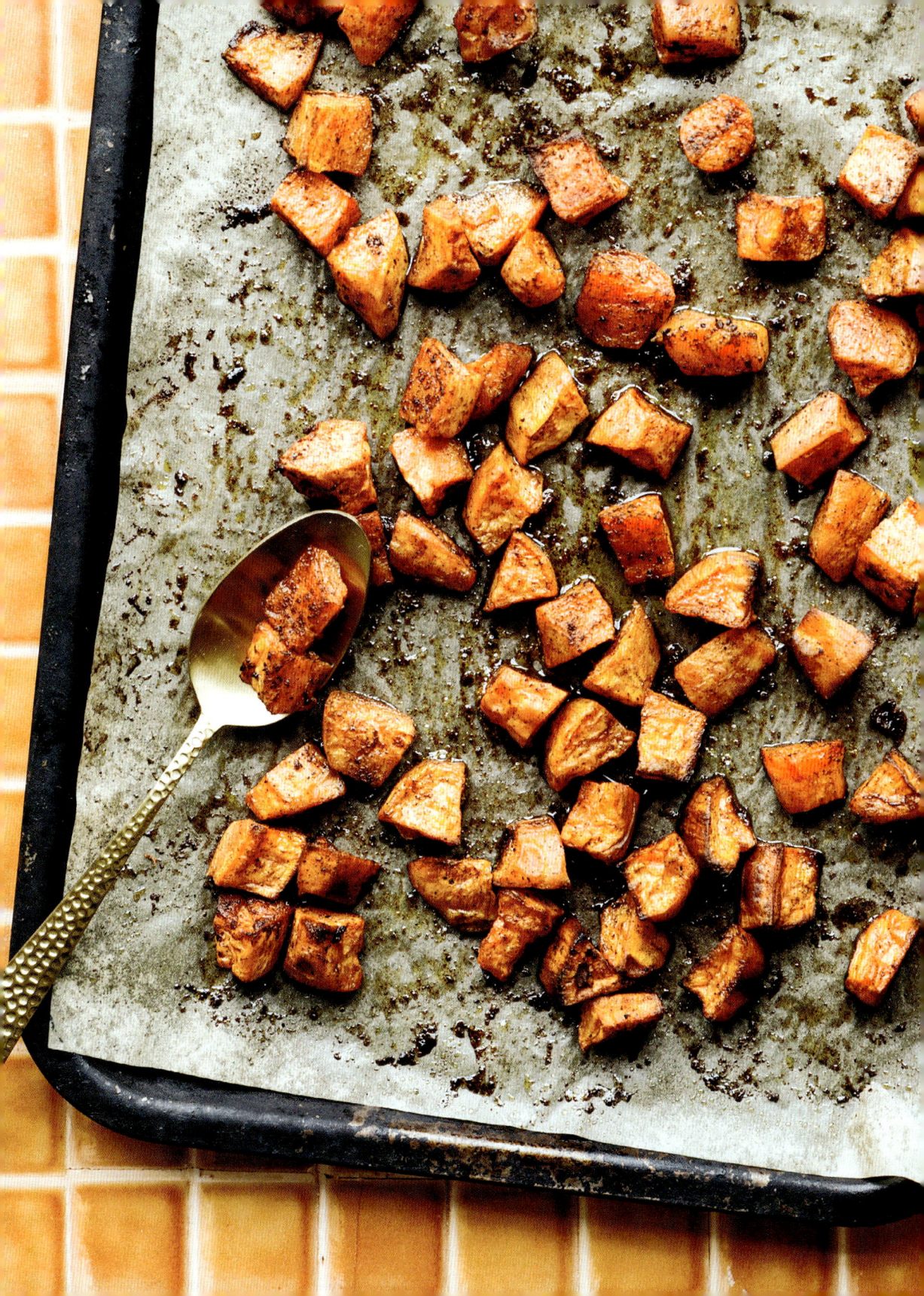

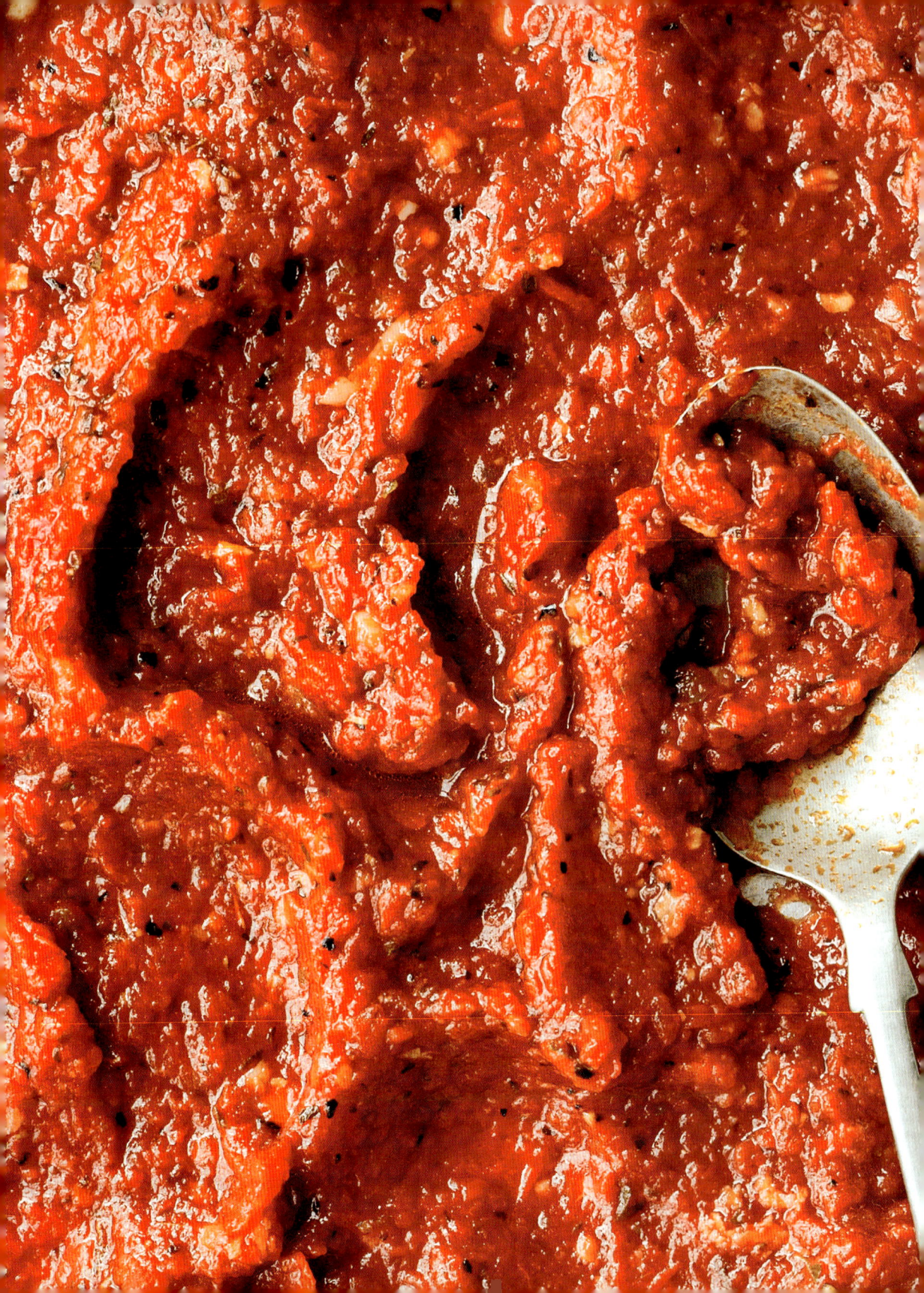

Homemade Marinara Dipping Sauce

I wanted to make sure that I included a tomato-based dip option in this cookbook since young kids often love tomato ketchup and are more willing to try new foods that look familiar to them. This dip has much greater depth of flavor than tomato ketchup, and more texture too, but is still bursting with that familiar rich tomato flavor. It's a great way to gently encourage toddlers to explore a wider variety of vegetables, which they can use as a dipper. If you think your toddler isn't ready for a more textured dip, feel free to use passata (sieved tomatoes) instead of canned finely chopped tomatoes (or crushed tomatoes), but you may need to cook it down for longer to get a thick dip. The maple syrup does a great job of balancing out the acidity of the tomatoes, but you can omit it for toddlers under 2 years old if you wish.

Serves:
Makes 1 cup (240 ml)

Prep Time:
5 minutes

Cook Time:
15 minutes

INGREDIENTS

1 tbsp (15 ml) avocado or olive oil

2 garlic cloves, minced

½ tsp onion granules or powder

1 tsp dried oregano

1 (15 oz [400 g]) can finely chopped tomatoes or crushed tomatoes (see notes)

1 tbsp (15 ml) balsamic vinegar

2 tsp (10 ml) pure maple syrup (optional for kids 2+ years)

Salt and black pepper, to taste

METHOD

Heat a small pan over medium heat and add the avocado oil. Once the oil is hot, add the minced garlic, onion granules and dried oregano and cook for 30 seconds, stirring continuously. Add the finely chopped tomatoes, balsamic vinegar, maple syrup, salt and black pepper and mix until well combined. Bring to a boil, turn the heat down to low and simmer uncovered for 10 minutes, or until the sauce has thickened, stirring occasionally. Turn off the heat, cover and allow the sauce to cool a little before serving. This dip can be served warm or cold.

STORAGE & REHEATING

Store in an airtight container in the refrigerator for up to 5 days. To freeze, divide the dip into individual portions (if desired) and freeze for up to 3 months. Defrost the dip overnight in the refrigerator or alternatively, you can reheat the dip from frozen on the stove with a splash of water, breaking it up with a spoon as it warms through.

NOTES

For this recipe, I recommend using the best quality canned tomatoes your budget will allow. The better quality the canned tomatoes, the better the results will be. Cheaper varieties tend to be waterier and more acidic and may change the consistency or texture of the dip.

30 READY IN 30 MINUTES OR LESS

MAKE-AHEAD

FREEZER FRIENDLY

VEGAN

SOMETHING DIFFERENT ON THE SIDE

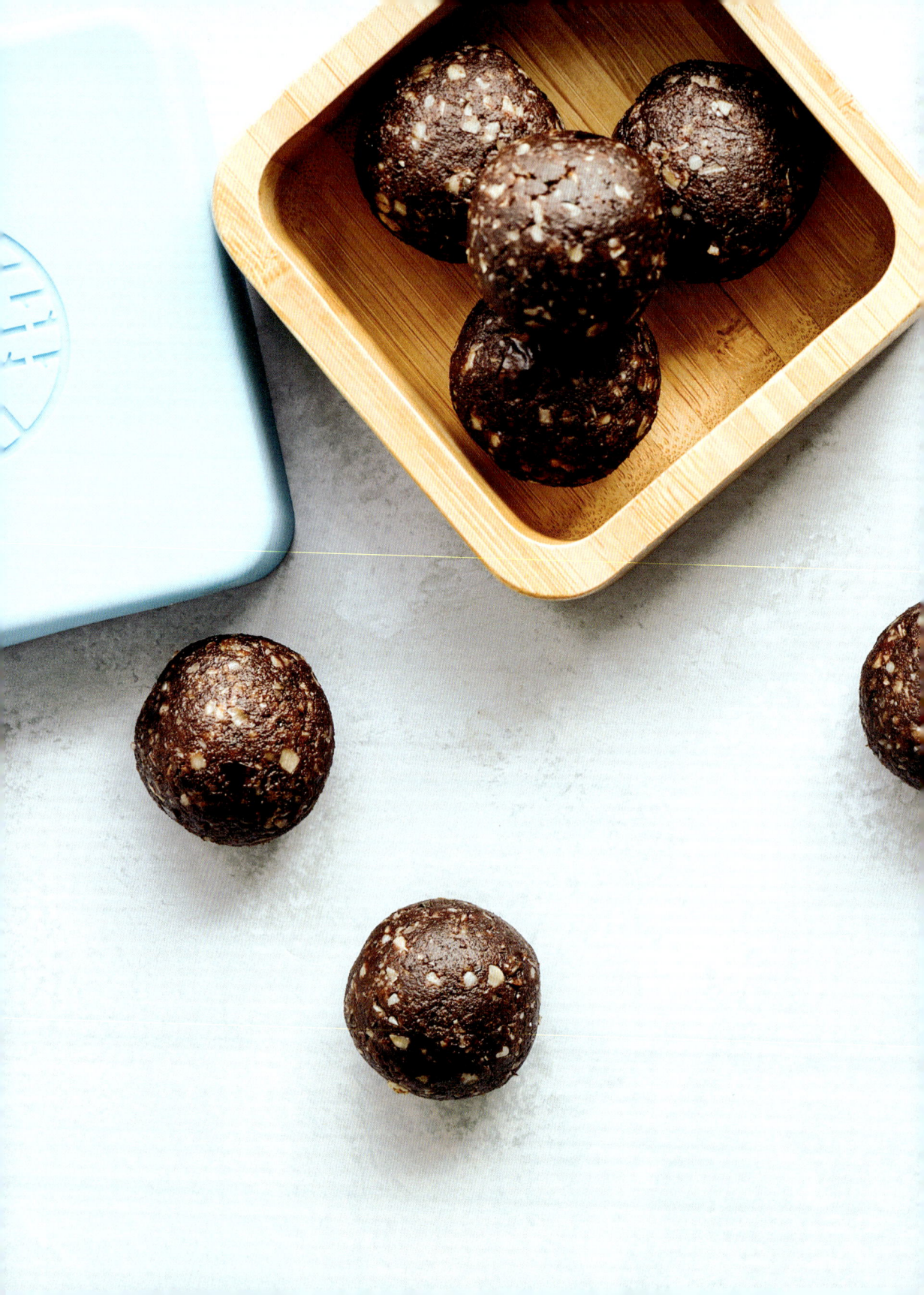

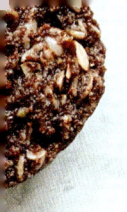

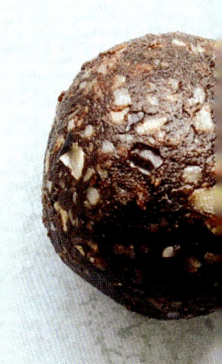

CHAPTER 6

Make-Ahead Snacks & Bakes

You can never have enough muffin and snack recipes, and this chapter doesn't disappoint! These recipes are great for batch cooking in advance for quick and easy snack options, and they also make for great breakfasts too. This is also a great opportunity to get your toddlers involved in cooking, as the recipes are super simple and easy to pull together.

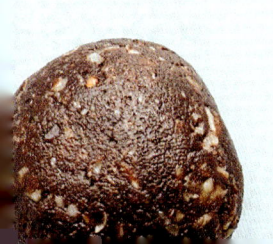

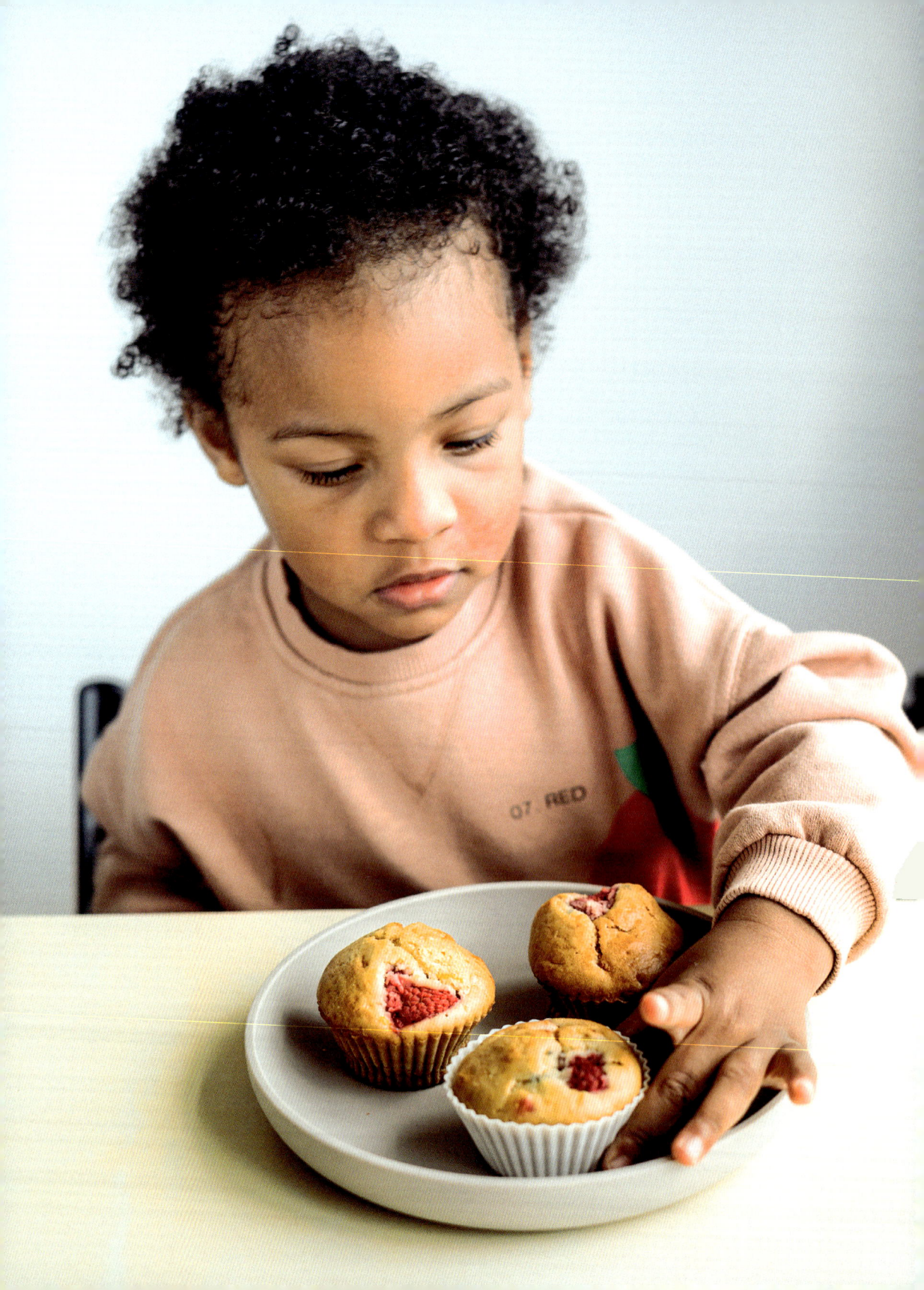

Orange & Raspberry Muffins

The absolute perfect light and fluffy fruity muffins, these never last long in our house! When cooking with raspberries, we typically reach for lemon as a complementary flavor, but orange also works incredibly well, and you'll wonder why you hadn't tried this combo before! If you want to add some fiber, you can do a 50/50 mix of all-purpose flour and whole-wheat flour, but just be aware that the texture of the muffin won't be as fluffy. Additionally, I do feel that the honey is essential here, and as such, I would recommend these muffins for kids aged 2 years and older—but as always, a few bites for younger toddlers won't hurt!

Serves: Makes 12 muffins

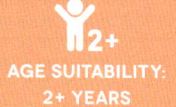

Prep Time: 10 minutes

Cook Time: 18 to 20 minutes

INGREDIENTS

Nonstick cooking spray, as needed

½ cup (120 ml) full-fat milk

2 large eggs

2 tbsp (30 ml) runny honey (see notes)

¼ cup (60 ml) melted unsalted butter

1 tsp pure vanilla extract

Zest of 1 medium-sized orange

¼ cup (60 ml) freshly squeezed orange juice

1½ cups (190 g) all-purpose flour

1 tsp baking powder

½ tsp baking soda

¼ tsp salt

1 cup (120 g) fresh or frozen raspberries

METHOD

Preheat the oven to 375°F (190°C, gas mark 5, fan 170°C) and line a 12-cup muffin tray with muffin cases, or spray it generously with the nonstick cooking spray.

In a medium bowl, add the milk, eggs, honey, melted butter, vanilla extract, orange zest and orange juice and whisk until well combined. In a separate large bowl, add the flour, baking powder, baking soda and salt and mix to combine.

Add the wet ingredients to the bowl of dry ingredients and mix until just combined—do not overmix the batter; a few lumps are okay. Add the raspberries and gently fold them into the batter.

Divide the batter evenly among the muffin cups. Bake the muffins for 18 to 20 minutes, or until they are golden and a toothpick inserted into the center of a muffin comes out clean of wet batter. Allow the muffins to cool slightly before removing them from the baking tray and cooling on a wire rack.

STORAGE & REHEATING

Store the muffins in an airtight container on the countertop for up to 3 days, or in the refrigerator for up to 5 days. To freeze the muffins, place the cooled muffins in a freezer bag in an even layer and freeze them for up to 3 months. Thaw them in the refrigerator or at room temperature. The frozen muffins can also be packed in a lunchbox, and they will thaw in 1 to 2 hours.

NOTES

Honey should never be given to babies under 12 months, even when cooked. This is due to the risk of infant botulism.

30 READY IN 30 MINUTES OR LESS

MAKE-AHEAD

FREEZER FRIENDLY

LUNCHBOX FRIENDLY

VEGETARIAN

ALLERGEN: DAIRY & EGG

2+ AGE SUITABILITY: 2+ YEARS

MAKE-AHEAD SNACKS & BAKES

Serves:
Makes 12 bars

Prep Time:
10 minutes +
4 hours to freeze

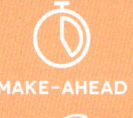

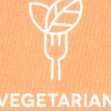

MAKE-AHEAD

VEGETARIAN

SOURCE OF FIBER, HEALTHY FATS, IRON & PROTEIN

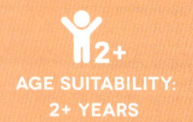

2+
AGE SUITABILITY:
2+ YEARS

No-Bake Multigrain Cereal Bars

My kids have always loved the cereal bars you get from the store, but they get super excited when they can join me in the kitchen to create our own version at home. What's more, it's the perfect opportunity to ramp up the nutrition and get some extra goodness into their growing bodies. These bars are jam packed with iron, protein and healthy fats! But the best thing here is that you don't need to bake them. The trouble with a lot of no-bake cereal bars is that they often fall apart when handled, but I figured out that freezing them is the key to holding their shape, and the addition of applesauce helps to keep the texture of the cereal soft enough for toddlers to eat. Due to the addition of honey (which counts as an added sugar), I'd recommend these bars for toddlers aged 2 years and older, but a few bites before then won't hurt!

INGREDIENTS

1½ cups (45 g) multigrain hoops cereal

1½ cups (45 g) puffed rice or rice snaps/crispies

¼ cup (30 g) ground flaxseed

½ cup (125 g) smooth peanut butter or sunflower seed butter

2 tbsp (30 ml) clear runny honey (see notes)

1 tsp pure vanilla extract

¼ cup (60 g) unsweetened applesauce (see notes)

METHOD

Line an 8 x 8-inch (20 x 20-cm) baking dish (see notes) with parchment paper and set aside.

In a large bowl, combine the multigrain hoops, puffed rice and ground flaxseed. Set aside.

Heat a small saucepan over low heat and add the peanut butter, honey and vanilla extract. Cook for 1 to 2 minutes, stirring the whole time, until the mixture becomes runny and easy to stir.

Add the wet mixture to the bowl of dry ingredients. Add the applesauce and using a wooden spoon, gently mix everything together until all the cereal is coated—this may take a couple of minutes to come together, but it gets easier the more you stir.

Transfer the mixture to the lined baking dish and using the back of the wooden spoon, spread the mixture out evenly and press it down gently but firmly. Keep pressing down until the mixture is tightly compacted in the baking dish—a loosely packed mixture will result in bars that crumble and fall apart, so don't skip this step!

Pop the baking dish in the freezer and freeze for at least 4 hours. Remove from the freezer and cut into 12 bars.

(Continued)

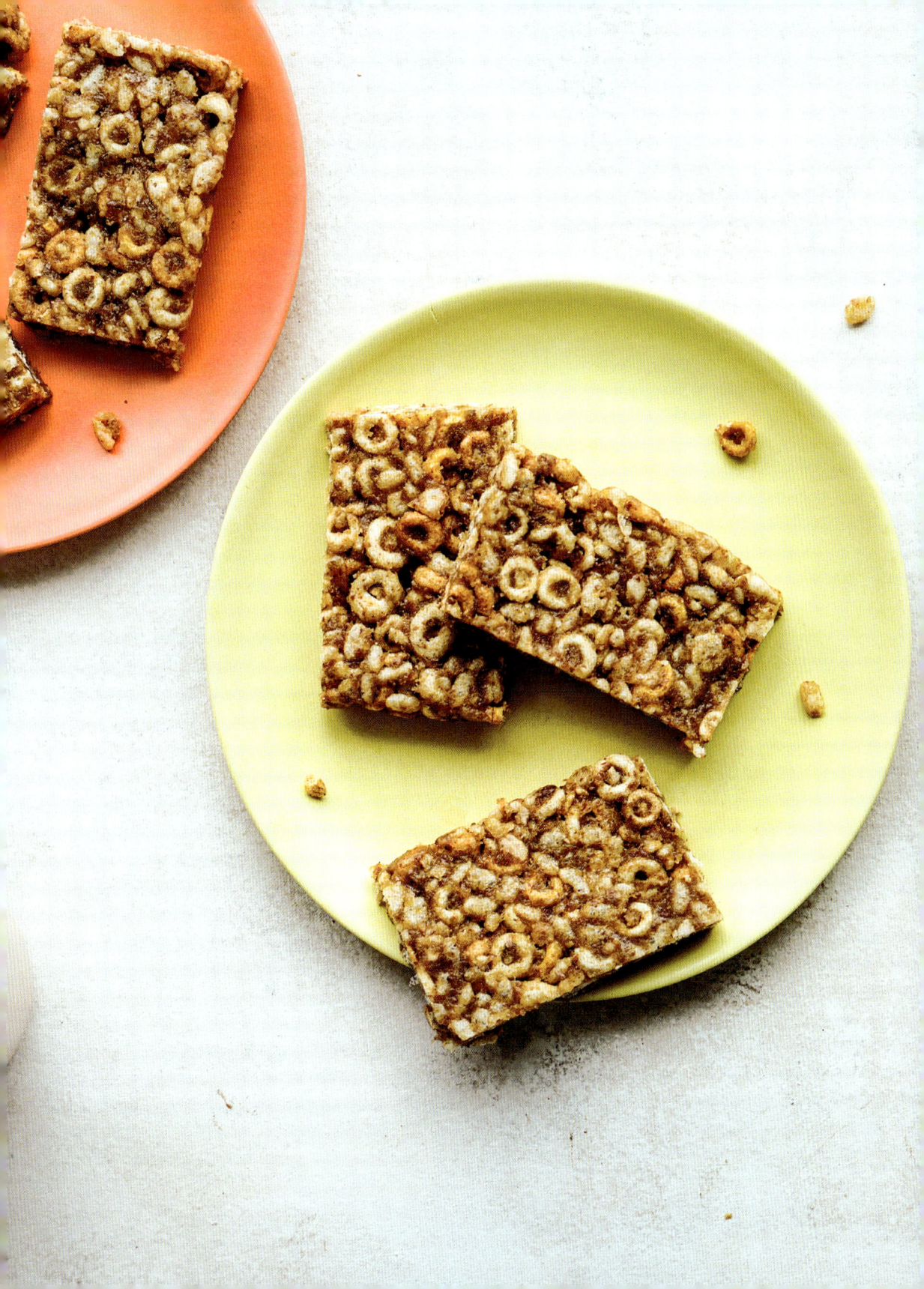

No-Bake Multigrain Cereal Bars (continued)

STORAGE

Stack the bars between sheets of parchment paper in a freezer bag and keep the bars in the freezer. To serve, remove a bar from the freezer and allow to stand for 5 to 10 minutes before eating. If you don't mind a crumblier, softer bar, you can store them in the refrigerator in an airtight container for up 5 days.

NOTES

If you are in the United Kingdom, please note that the applesauce referenced in this recipe is pureed apples, not the chunky applesauce you typically find in the condiment section at the supermarket. Applesauce is now widely available in the U.K, but if you're having trouble finding it, be sure to check out the baby aisle for the apple puree pouches, which are the same thing, just in smaller quantities.

Honey should never be given to babies under 12 months, even when cooked. This is due to the risk of infant botulism.

I have listed the size of the baking dish I use at home, but feel free to use whichever size baking dish or tray you have on hand—as long it's approximately medium size, it will work.

Bite-Size Fruity Cheesecake Strudels

I always make sure I have a packet of ready rolled pastry on hand for when we feel like a quick and easy treat, and these Bite-Size Fruity Cheesecake Strudels are perfect for little hands. I always have a crowd around me when I make these, and it's easy to understand why—sweet berries coupled with comforting cream cheese and wrapped in a gorgeously golden and flaky pastry. It's a match made in heaven! The addition of chia seeds not only gives a boost of iron and protein, but also gives the berries a jammy texture, which helps it to stay in place as the pastry cooks.

INGREDIENTS

1 cup (120 g) fresh or thawed frozen raspberries or strawberries

2 tsp (7 g) dried chia seeds

½ cup (120 g) full-fat cream cheese

1 tbsp (15 ml) pure maple syrup (optional for kids 2+ years)

½ tsp vanilla extract

1 (9 x 14–inch [23 x 35–cm]) sheet frozen rolled puff pastry, thawed (see notes)

1 egg, whisked (see notes for egg-free option)

METHOD

Preheat the oven to 400°F (200°C, gas mark 6, fan 180°C) and line a large baking sheet with parchment paper.

Add the raspberries to a medium bowl and mash them with a fork. Add the chia seeds and mix until well combined. Set aside.

In a separate small bowl, add the cream cheese, maple syrup (if using) and vanilla extract and cream until light and fluffy. Set aside.

Gently unroll the thawed puff pastry sheet onto a dry surface or chopping board and use a sharp knife to roughly cut sixteen rectangles. Making sure the rectangles are positioned lengthwise, make three small cuts into one half of each rectangle so that the steam can escape during cooking.

Distribute the cream cheese mixture on the other half of each rectangle (opposite the cuts), being careful not to overfill. Add a small dollop of the raspberry and chia seed mixture on top of the cream cheese mixture on each rectangle and carefully fold the pastry over so that side with the cuts covers the top of the raspberry and cream cheese. Use a fork to gently press and seal the edges and transfer each strudel to the lined baking sheet.

Using a pastry brush, brush the strudels with the whisked egg, making sure all the visible pastry is coated. Bake in the oven for 20 to 25 minutes, or until golden brown and puffed.

(Continued)

Serves:
Makes 16 bite-size strudels

Prep Time:
10 minutes

Cook Time:
20 to 25 minutes

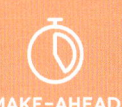

MAKE-AHEAD

FREEZER FRIENDLY

LUNCHBOX FRIENDLY

VEGETARIAN

ALLERGEN: DAIRY

SOURCE OF IRON & PROTEIN

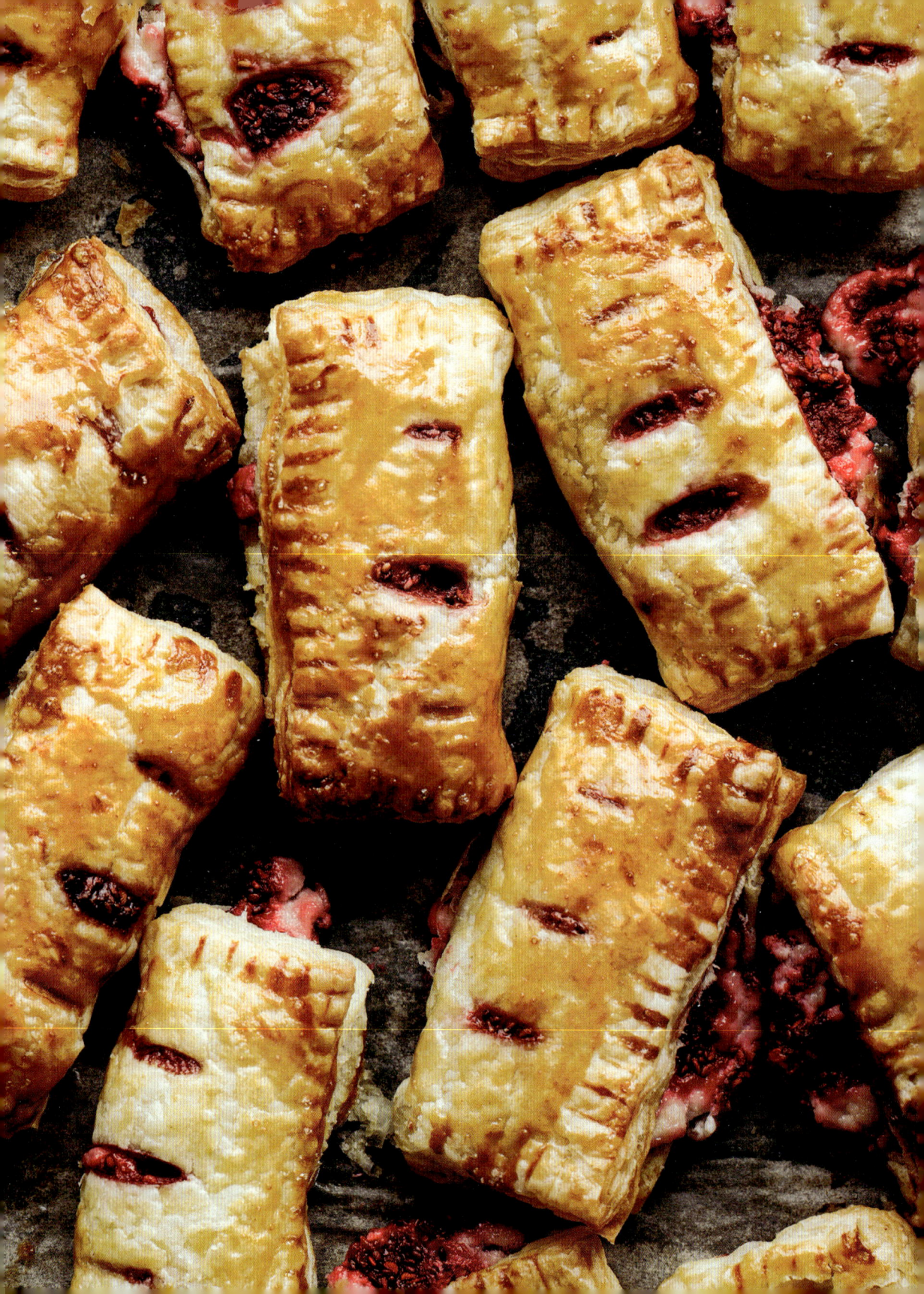

Bite-Size Fruity Cheesecake Strudels (continued)

STORAGE & REHEATING
Store the strudels in an airtight container in the refrigerator for up to 3 days. To freeze them, arrange the cooled strudels on a large baking sheet and flash-freeze them for 1 hour. Transfer the strudels to a freezer bag and keep them in the freezer for up to 3 months. To reheat from frozen, place the strudels on a large lined baking sheet and bake them in the oven at 350°F (180°C, gas mark 4, fan 160°C) for 15 to 20 minutes or until warmed through.

NOTES
If you are in the United Kingdom, note that the puff pastry listed in this recipe is equal to 1 (11-oz [312-g]) packet of frozen puff pastry.

If your toddler has an egg allergy, you can substitute the egg wash with the milk of your choice.

Serves:
Makes 12 cookies

Prep Time:
10 minutes

Cook Time:
10 to 15 minutes

30 READY IN 30 MINUTES OR LESS

MAKE-AHEAD

LUNCHBOX FRIENDLY

VEGAN

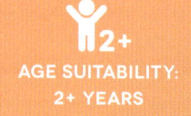

ALLERGEN: NUTS

SOURCE OF FIBER, HEALTHY FATS, IRON & PROTEIN

2+ AGE SUITABILITY: 2+ YEARS

Iron-Rich Almond & Coconut Cookies

I've been working on this cookie recipe for some time now because I wanted to make sure that I struck a good balance between getting the cookie texture soft enough for younger toddlers, while also maintaining that classic cookie likeness for older toddlers who have likely sampled a cookie or two by now. These cookies are chewy and decadent on the inside, and crisp and golden on the outside, but not super crunchy in their entirety, which could scratch sensitive teething gums. The best part is they require such simple ingredients, and the almond and coconut flavors are reminiscent of coconut macaroons. The almond meal in particular is a fantastic source of iron and protein. One quick tip: Don't be tempted to overcook these cookies in an attempt to make them uniformly golden. It's just the edges that need color, with the rest of the cookie retaining its milky, creamy hue.

INGREDIENTS

- 1¼ cups (125 g) almond meal (see notes)
- ½ cup (50 g) unsweetened shredded or desiccated coconut
- ½ tsp baking powder
- 2 tbsp (30 ml) melted coconut oil, cooled
- 2 tbsp (30 ml) pure maple syrup
- ½ tsp pure vanilla extract
- ½ tsp almond extract

NOTES
Almond meal is also known as ground almonds and is typically found in the baking section at the grocery store.

METHOD

Preheat the oven to 350°F (180°C, gas mark 4, fan 160°C) and line a large baking tray with parchment paper.

In a medium bowl, combine the almond meal, shredded coconut and baking powder. In a separate small bowl, add the cooled melted coconut oil, maple syrup, vanilla extract and almond extract and whisk to combine. Add the wet ingredients to the bowl of dry ingredients, and using a wooden spoon, mix until well combined.

Use your hands to gently knead the dough—the warmth from your hand will release the oils from the almond meal and help the dough to form.

Shape the mixture into ball shapes, using 1 tablespoon (15 g) of the mixture for each ball. If the dough is slightly crumbly, you can gently squeeze and press the mixture together to help form a ball shape before rolling.

Arrange the balls a couple of inches apart on the prepared baking sheet. Use a fork to gently press down on each ball to flatten them. The balls may slightly crack when flattened, and this is okay—the cracks will become golden and crunchy and complement the cookie once baked.

Bake for 10 to 15 minutes, or until the edges start to turn golden. The cookies will harden as they cool but will still retain a chewy texture in the center.

STORAGE
Store in an airtight container for up to 5 days.

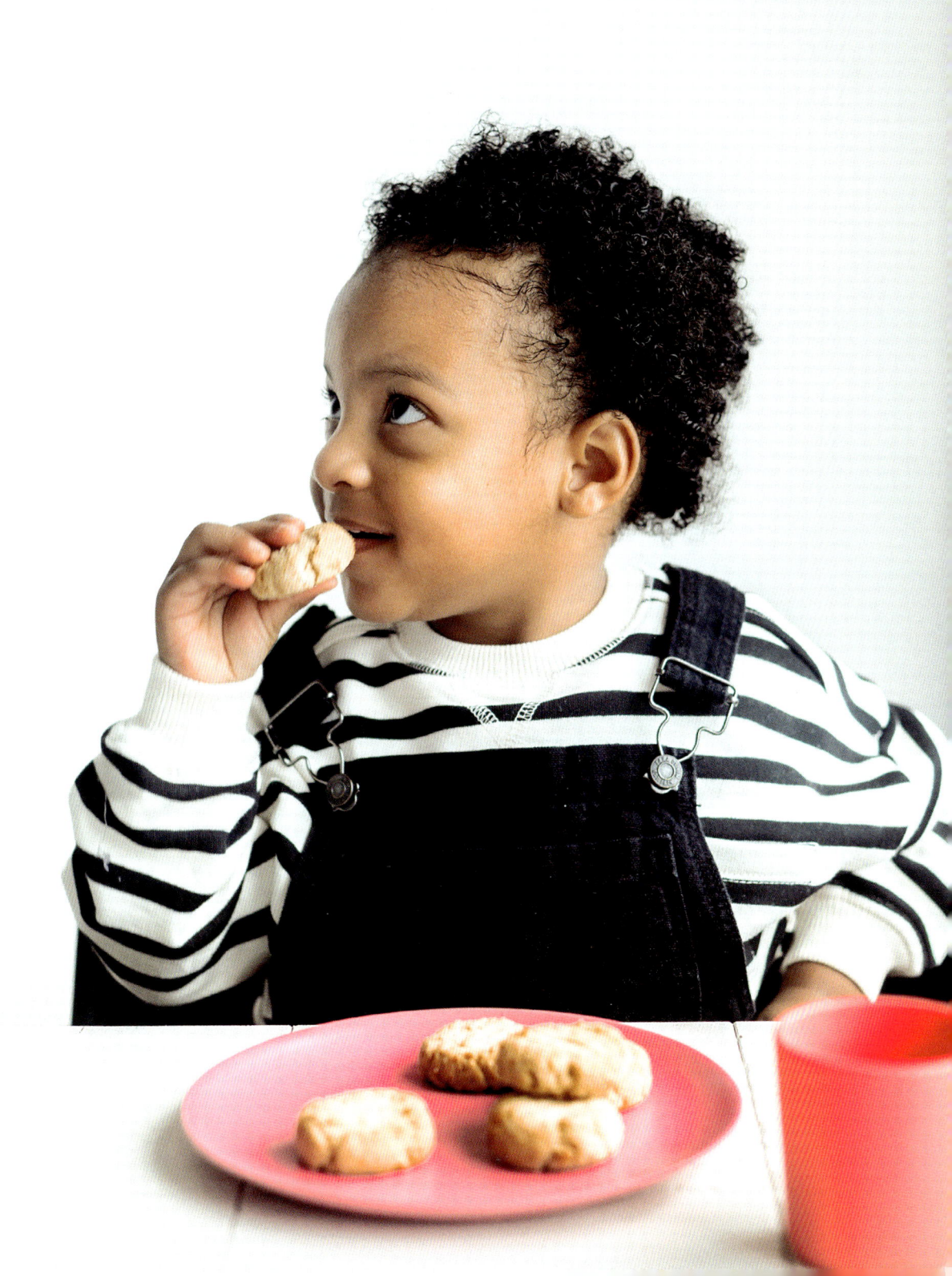

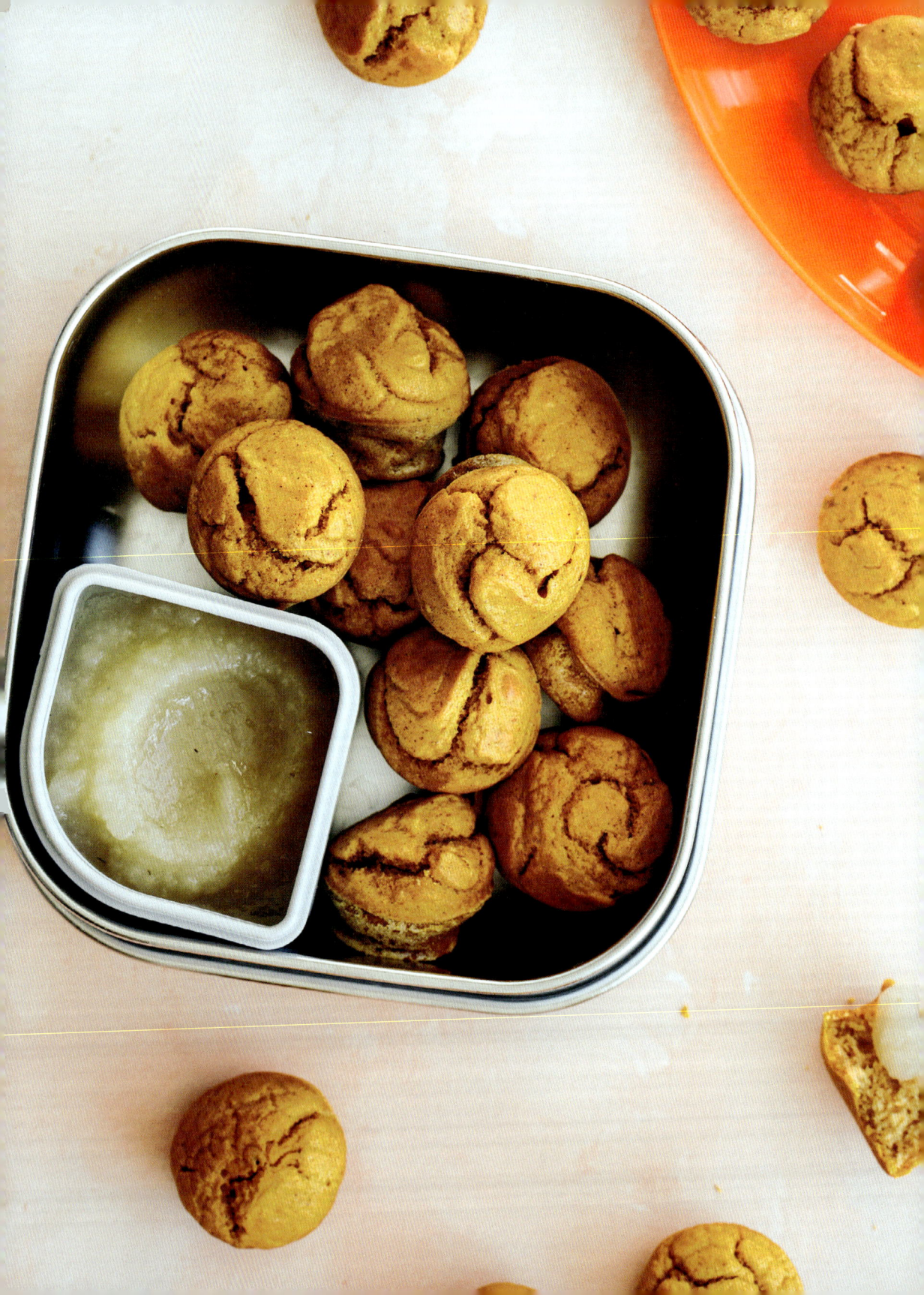

Pumpkin Pie Mini Muffins

You've probably noticed by now that my blender makes a regular appearance when I'm baking and that's because it saves so much time and creates significantly less washing up, which is always my goal. This recipe is probably the easiest of them all, and it comes together in less than 20 minutes! The muffins themselves are light, soft and enveloped in the deliciously warming spiced flavors of fall—but of course, they can be enjoyed at any time of the year. The mini size works so perfectly here, as not only is it the perfect size for little hands, but it also helps to keep the muffins moist. Mini muffin pans are widely available and are very affordable—I've seen the silicone variety (which I prefer for this size) at the dollar store.

Serves:
Makes 24 mini muffins

Prep Time:
5 minutes

Cook Time:
10 to 12 minutes

INGREDIENTS

Nonstick cooking spray, as needed

1 cup (125 g) all-purpose flour

1 tsp baking powder

½ tsp baking soda

1 tsp pumpkin spice (see notes)

½ cup (125 g) canned pumpkin puree

¾ cup (180 ml) cow's milk or nondairy milk of choice

1 large egg

1 tbsp (15 ml) melted butter or coconut oil, slightly cooled

2 tbsp (30 ml) maple syrup (optional for kids 2+ years)

1 tsp pure vanilla extract

METHOD

Preheat the oven to 375°F (190°C, gas mark 5, fan 170°C) and line a 24-cup mini muffin tray with muffin cases, or spray the tray generously with the nonstick cooking spray.

Add the flour, baking powder, baking soda, pumpkin spice, pumpkin puree, milk, egg, butter, maple syrup (if using) and vanilla extract into a blender and blend on high speed for 30 seconds. Remove the blender lid, scrape down the sides and blend again until the batter is smooth—a few lumps are okay.

Distribute the batter evenly among the muffin cups and bake for approximately 10 to 12 minutes, or until a toothpick inserted into the center of a muffin comes out clean of wet batter. Allow to cool completely before turning out.

STORAGE & REHEATING

Store the muffins in an airtight container in the refrigerator for up to 3 days. To freeze the muffins, place the cooled muffins in a freezer bag in an even layer and freeze them for up to 3 months. Thaw them in the refrigerator or at room temperature. Frozen muffins can be packed in a lunchbox and will thaw in 1 to 2 hours.

NOTES

If you don't have pumpkin spice mix, you can substitute 1 teaspoon of ground cinnamon and ½ teaspoon of ground nutmeg.

READY IN 30 MINUTES OR LESS

MAKE-AHEAD

FREEZER FRIENDLY

LUNCHBOX FRIENDLY

VEGETARIAN

ALLERGEN: EGG

Serves:
Makes 12 to 16 balls

Prep Time:
5 minutes

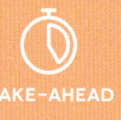

Cook Time:
45 minutes

MAKE-AHEAD

FREEZER FRIENDLY

LUNCHBOX FRIENDLY

VEGETARIAN

ALLERGEN: DAIRY & EGG

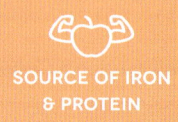

SOURCE OF IRON & PROTEIN

Cheesy Broccoli Balls

The perfect nutritious snack that is great for lunchboxes, these mini savory balls are crispy, fluffy, cheesy and comforting, and they freeze beautifully! Such a great way to experiment with serving broccoli too, which provides subtle flavor without being intimidating or overpowering. But the best parts are the chickpeas and cheese because, between them, they add a glorious dose of iron, protein and staying power—meaning these little balls will keep kids fuller for longer! And of course, they are not just for kids. I adore these as a hearty snack or appetizer with my Homemade Marinara Dipping Sauce (page 127) on the side.

INGREDIENTS

5¾ cups (525 g) broccoli florets

1 (14-oz [400-g]) can chickpeas, drained and rinsed

1 cup (60 g) panko breadcrumbs

1 cup (115 g) grated cheddar cheese

1 tsp garlic granules or powder

1 tsp dried parsley

2 scallions (white and green parts), finely chopped

2 large eggs

Salt and black pepper, to taste

Nonstick cooking spray, as needed

METHOD

Preheat the oven to 400°F (200°C, gas mark 6, fan 180°C) and line a baking sheet with parchment paper.

Bring a large pot of water to boil over high heat and add the broccoli florets. Boil for 10 to 15 minutes, or until fork tender. Once the broccoli is cooked, drain the water thoroughly. Alternatively, you can steam the broccoli for 15 to 17 minutes, or until fork tender.

Meanwhile, mash the drained chickpeas with a fork and add them to a large bowl. Add the panko breadcrumbs, grated cheese, garlic granules, dried parsley, chopped scallions, eggs, salt and black pepper and mix until everything is well combined. Set aside.

Roughly chop the cooked broccoli florets and gently fold them into the mixture until well combined. Shape the mixture into ball shapes, using 2 tablespoons (30 g) of the mixture for each ball, and arrange the balls on the prepared baking sheet. Spray generously with the nonstick cooking spray and bake for 18 to 20 minutes, or until they are golden. Allow the balls to cool slightly before using a spatula to gently ease them off the baking sheet.

STORAGE & REHEATING

Store leftovers in an airtight container in the refrigerator for up to 3 days. To freeze, arrange the cooled balls on a baking sheet and flash-freeze them for 1 hour. Transfer them to a freezer bag and keep them in the freezer for up to 3 months.

Thaw in the refrigerator overnight and serve cold or reheat in the microwave covered on the high setting in 30-second intervals until warmed through. The frozen balls can be packed in a lunchbox and will thaw in 1 to 2 hours.

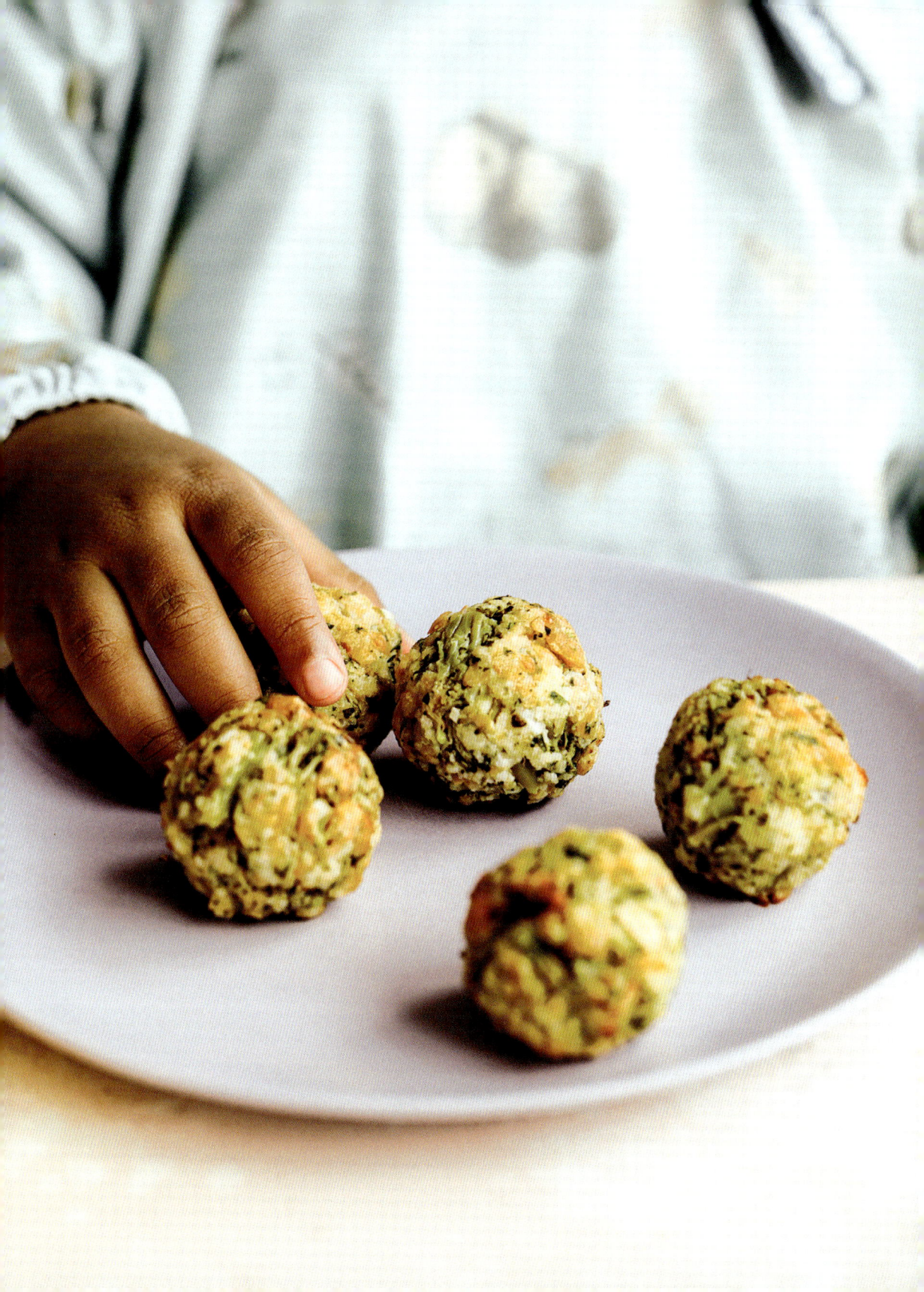

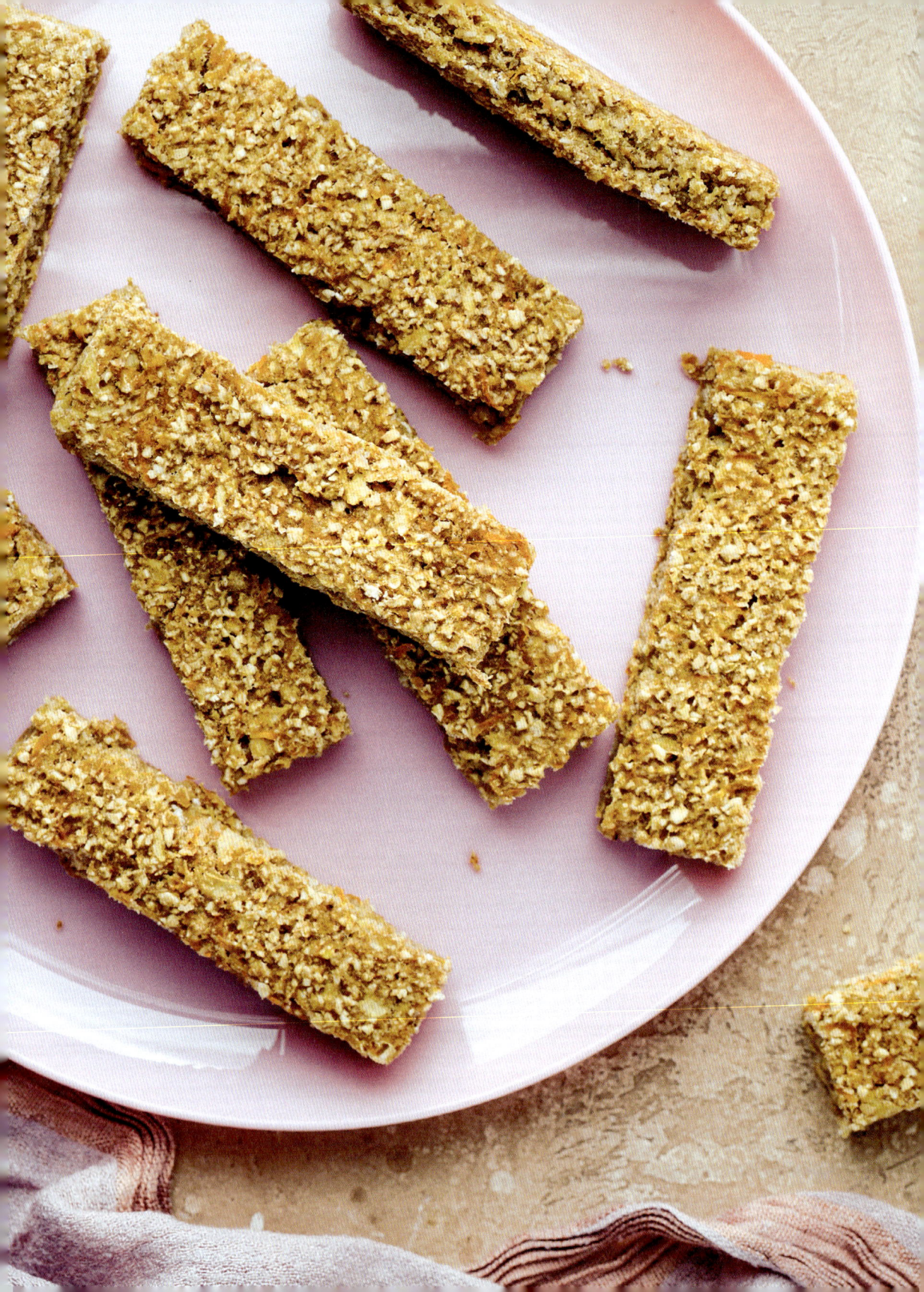

Apple & Carrot Snack Bars

Kids tend to love oat bars, and this recipe ticks all the boxes for a toddler-friendly, tasty and nutritious snack. The bars come together quickly and easily, and they are naturally sweetened with banana and apple, without any added sugars at all! You can add a splash of maple syrup or honey if you fancy, but your toddler won't notice if you don't. The best thing about these bars is the texture—they are soft and easy to eat, which is a huge plus if your little one is teething, but they are not mushy or crumbly, which means less mess! This recipe makes a big batch, so be sure to freeze half for quick and easy snacks as needed.

Serves:
Makes 16 mini bars

Prep Time:
10 minutes

Cook Time:
20 to 25 minutes

INGREDIENTS

2½ cups (225 g) rolled oats

2 medium apples, peeled, cored and roughly chopped

2 medium ripe bananas

1⅓ cup (140 g) shredded carrot

¼ cup (40 g) hemp hearts

1 tsp ground cinnamon

METHOD

Preheat the oven to 350°F (180°C, gas mark 4, fan 160°C) and line a 9 x 9-inch (23 x 23-cm) baking tray with parchment paper, ensuring some of the paper is draping over two sides of the tray.

Add the oats to a food processor and blend on high until the oats break down to a flour consistency. Transfer the blended oats to a large bowl and set aside.

Add the chopped apples and bananas to the same food processor and blend on high until you get a puree consistency. Add the puree to the bowl of blended oats, along with the shredded carrot, hemp hearts and cinnamon, and mix until combined.

Transfer the mixture to the lined baking tray and smooth it out with a spatula. Bake in the oven for 20 to 25 minutes, or until golden and bouncy to the touch. Allow to cool slightly before lifting it out of the baking tray to finish cooling on a wire rack. Once completely cooled, cut into mini bars and serve.

STORAGE

Store the bars in an airtight container in the refrigerator for up to 3 days or freeze for up to 3 months. Thaw the bars in the refrigerator or at room temperature, or alternatively in the microwave on the high setting for 20-second intervals until thawed. The frozen bars can also be packed in a lunchbox, and they will thaw in 1 to 2 hours.

NOTES

Feel free to use any similar-sized baking tray. The exact size doesn't matter, as it's a very forgiving recipe.

MAKE-AHEAD

FREEZER FRIENDLY

LUNCHBOX FRIENDLY

VEGAN

SOURCE OF FIBER, HEALTHY FATS, IRON & PROTEIN

Serves:
Makes 12 muffins

Prep Time:
10 minutes

Cook Time:
20 to 25 minutes

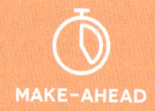

MAKE-AHEAD

FREEZER FRIENDLY

LUNCHBOX FRIENDLY

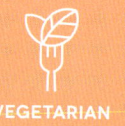

VEGETARIAN

ALLERGEN:
DAIRY & EGG

SOURCE OF PROTEIN

Lemon & Blueberry Yogurt Muffins

Everyone loves a good blueberry muffin, and my Lemon & Blueberry Yogurt Muffins are so popular on my Instagram page that I wanted to make sure I reserved a spot for them in this cookbook! These muffins are super soft and fluffy and bursting with zesty lemon citrus flavor, which complements the blueberries so well. The Greek yogurt provides just enough moisture without making them too heavy and adds a hearty dose of protein. I personally find these muffins are sweet enough without the maple syrup, but feel free to add in a couple of tablespoons if your blueberries aren't sweet enough to carry the load.

INGREDIENTS

Nonstick cooking spray

2 large eggs

1 cup (280 g) full-fat plain Greek yogurt

½ cup (120 ml) extra virgin olive oil

2 tbsp (12 g) lemon zest

¼ cup (60 ml) freshly squeezed lemon juice

2 tbsp (30 ml) pure maple syrup (optional for kids 2+ years)

1 tsp vanilla extract

2 cups (250 g) all-purpose flour

1 tsp baking powder

1 tsp baking soda

¼ tsp salt

¼ cup (60 ml) whole fat milk, if needed

1½ cups (225 g) blueberries (fresh or frozen)

METHOD

Preheat the oven to 375°F (190°C, gas mark 5, fan 170°C) and line a 12-cup muffin tray with silicone muffin cases or spray the tray generously with the nonstick cooking spray

In a large bowl, add the eggs and whisk for 2 minutes, until frothy. Add the yogurt, extra virgin olive oil, lemon zest, lemon juice, maple syrup (if using) and vanilla extract. Whisk again until smooth.

Add the flour, baking powder, baking soda and salt and mix until well combined. Depending on the thickness/brand of the Greek yogurt, you may need to add the milk to loosen up the batter. The batter is supposed to be thick and will have some lumps, so only add the milk if the batter is too thick to scoop into the muffin tray. Do not over mix as this will result in dry, dense muffins.

Gently fold in the blueberries until just combined and distribute the batter evenly among the muffin cups. Bake for approximately 20 to 25 minutes, or until a toothpick inserted into the center of a muffin comes out clean of wet batter. Transfer the muffins from the muffin pan to a wire rack to cool completely before serving.

STORAGE

Store the muffins in an airtight container in the refrigerator for up to 3 days. To freeze the muffins, place the cooled muffins in a freezer bag in an even layer and freeze them for up to 3 months. Thaw them in the refrigerator or at room temperature. Frozen muffins can be packed in a lunchbox and will thaw in 1 to 2 hours.

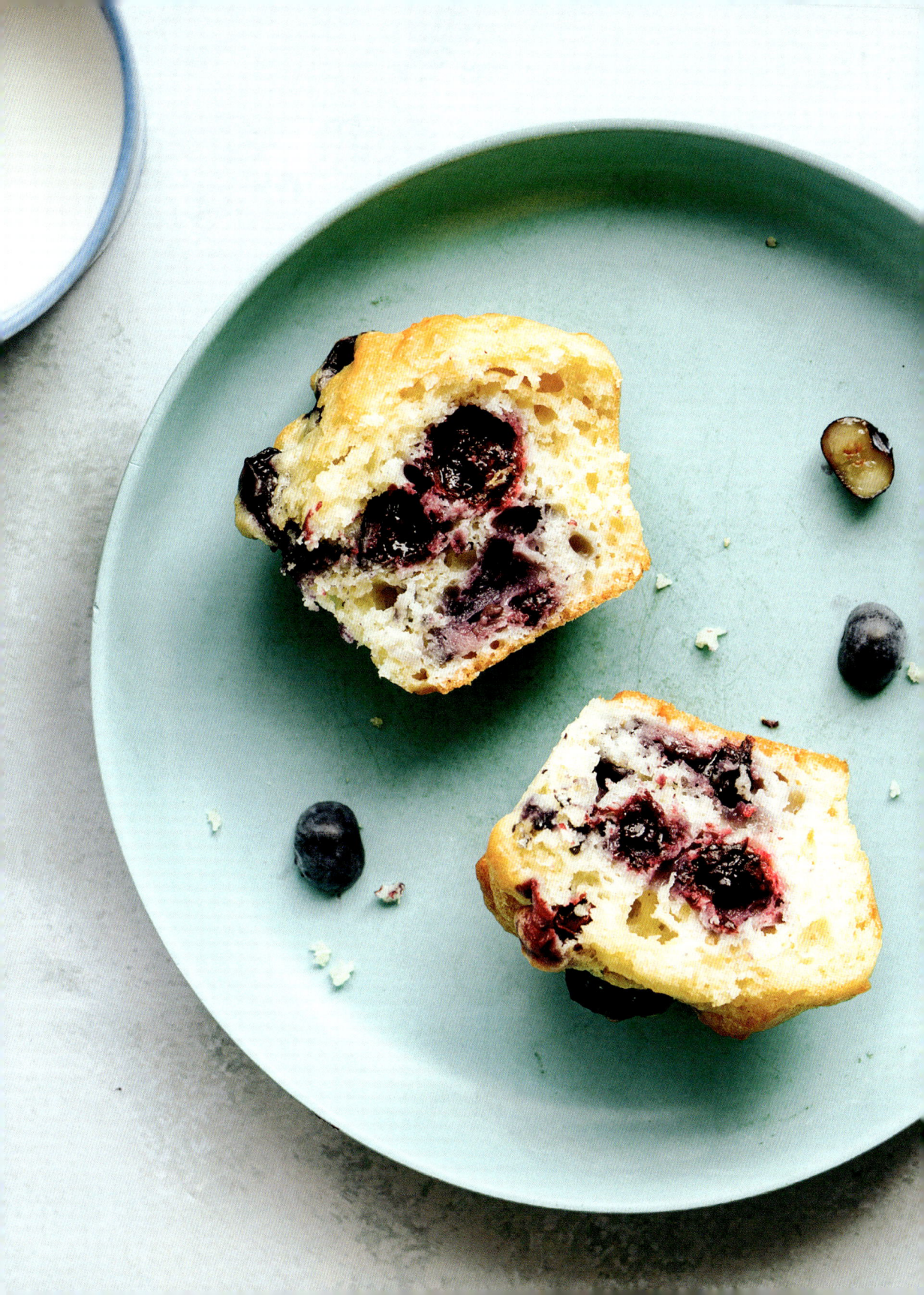

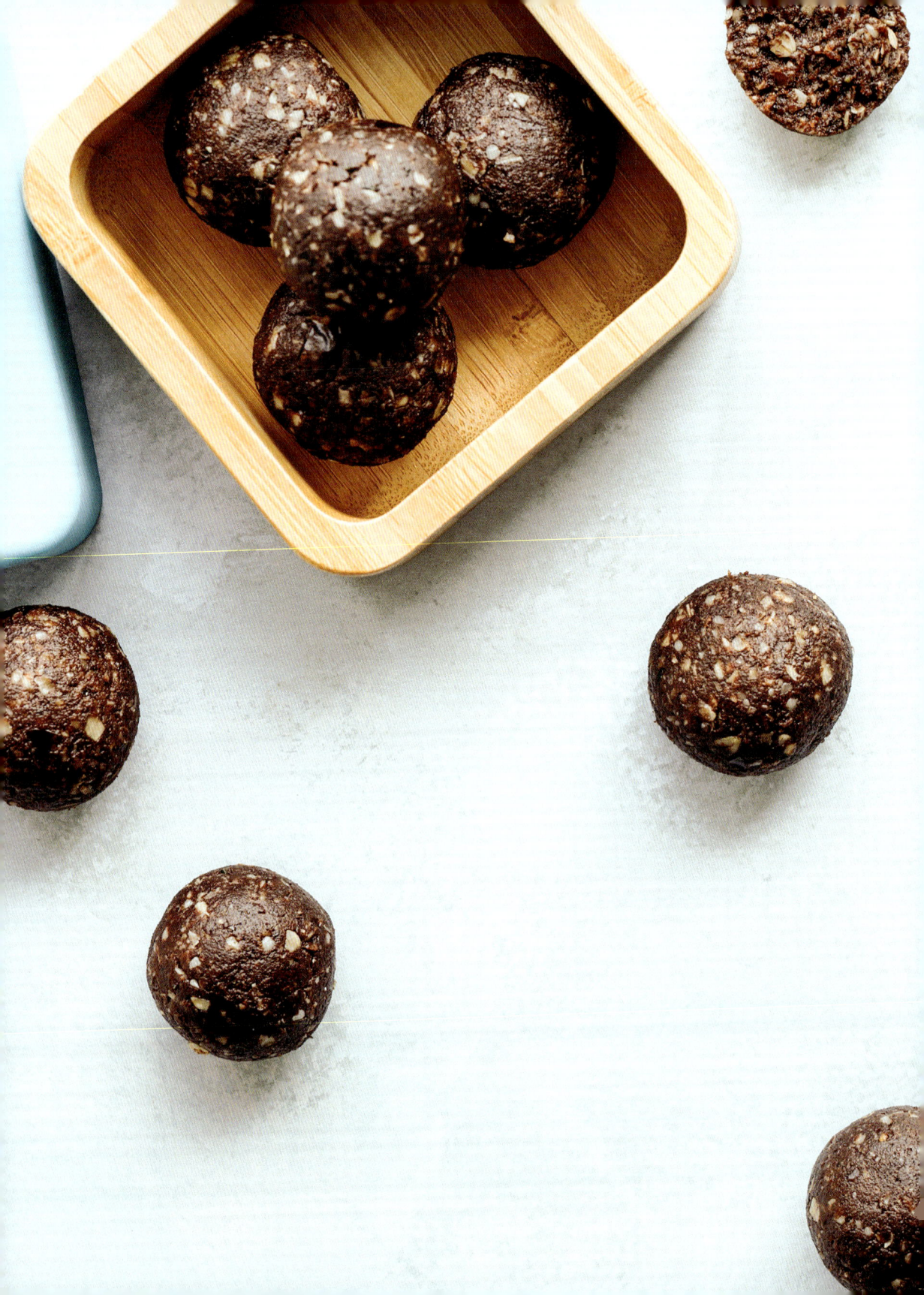

Chocolate Oat Bites

I love making foods that my kids salivate over, especially when the foods are absolutely full of goodness for their growing bodies. These chocolate oat bites tick both boxes! Nutritional powerhouses, as well as delightful morsels of fudgy chocolate deliciousness, they are such a wonderful dessert option! The medjool dates do a wonderful job of providing natural sweetness, with deep notes reminiscent of caramel, and the combination of fiber-packed oats and protein-packed peanut butter and hemp make these an exceptionally filling snack option too. Due to the cocoa powder, I do recommend that these are reserved for kids 2 years and older, and be sure to take extra care when brushing your toddler's teeth due to the generous helping of dates, which can stick to their teeth.

INGREDIENTS

8 medjool dates, pitted

1 cup (90 g) rolled oats

2 tbsp (20 g) hulled hemp hearts

3 tbsp (15 g) cocoa powder

¼ cup (65 g) smooth nut butter or seed butter of choice

¼ cup (60 ml) melted coconut oil, cooled

METHOD

To soften the pitted dates, place them in a bowl of boiling water for 5 minutes—do not skip this step, otherwise your oat balls will lack moisture and be dry and crumbly.

Meanwhile, add the rolled oats, hemp hearts, cocoa powder, nut butter and melted coconut oil to a food processor. Drain the pitted dates, add them to the food processor and blend on low speed for 1 to 2 minutes, until the mixture comes together.

Roll the mixture into ball shapes using 1 tablespoon (15 g) of the mixture for each ball and refrigerate for 1 hour before serving.

STORAGE & REHEATING

Store in an airtight container in the refrigerator for up to 5 days or freeze for up 1 month. Thaw them in the refrigerator or at room temperature. The frozen oat balls can also be packed in a lunchbox, and they will thaw in 1 to 2 hours.

Serves:
Makes 16–18 balls

Prep Time:
15 minutes + 1 hour to chill

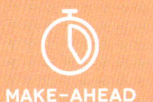

Cook Time:
10 minutes

MAKE-AHEAD

FREEZER FRIENDLY

LUNCHBOX FRIENDLY

VEGAN

SOURCE OF FIBER, HEALTHY FATS, IRON & PROTEIN

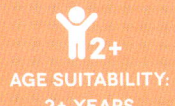

AGE SUITABILITY: 2+ YEARS

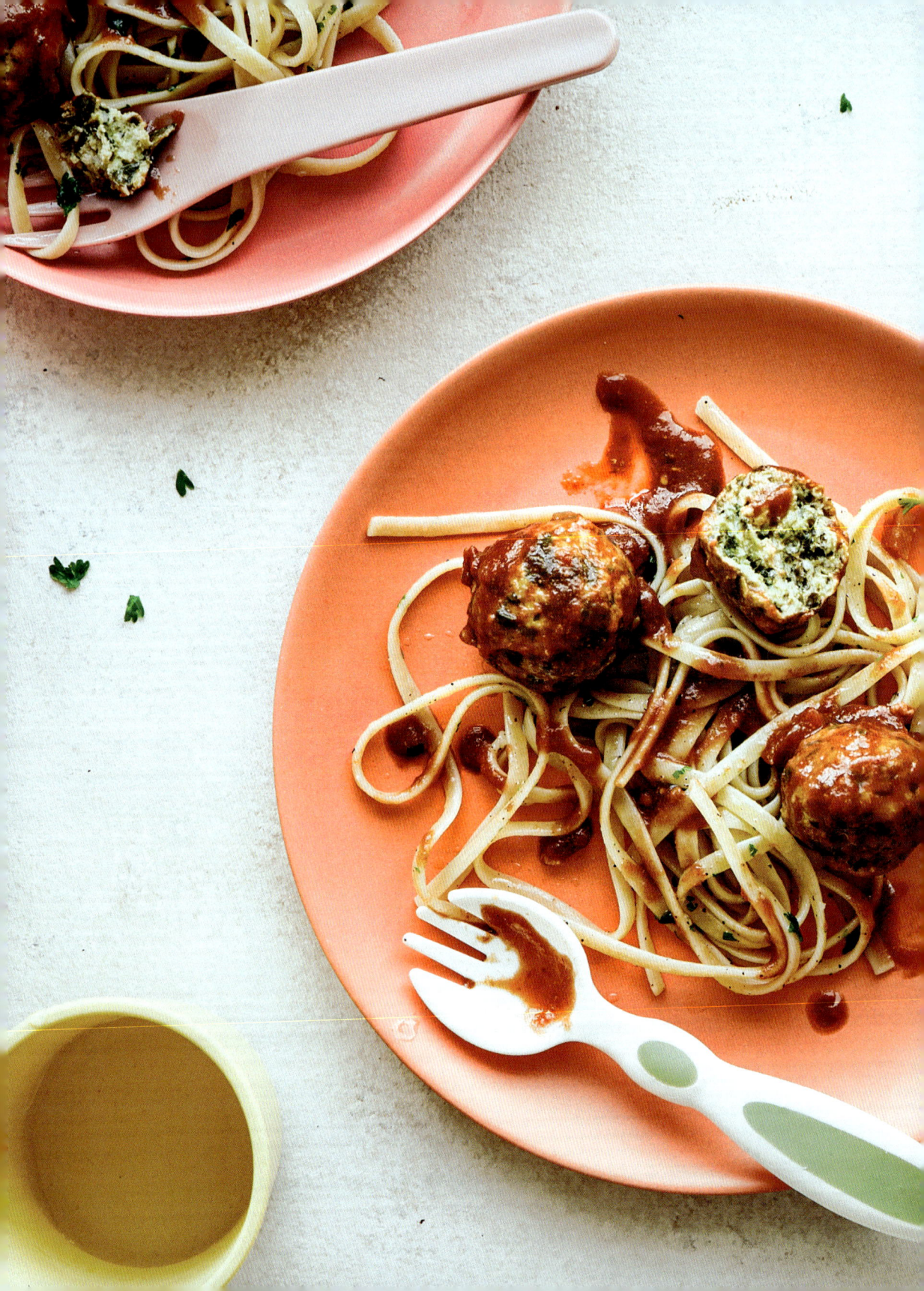

CHAPTER 7

Meal Plans

As we come to the end of this cookbook, I want to provide you with one last resource that will help you to incorporate the recipes from this book into your day-to-day lives. People often ask me how I manage to consistently cook nutritious and balanced meals for my family and how I am able to incorporate a wide variety of foods into my kids' diets. It boils down to two main things: batch cooking and meal plans, both of which will be utilized in this chapter! There's no doubt about it: It can feel very overwhelming and exhausting to think of and cook three meals a day, week in, week out, and try to keep things balanced and varied, especially on those busy mornings when you are rushing out of the door or at the end of a tiring day. This meal plan takes the stress out of that daily question of what to eat, helps you to stay organized and encourages you to make nutritious and varied home-cooked meals a reality.

Not everyone is into meal plans, and that's okay, but if you are feeling stuck in a rut or overwhelmed with thinking about day-to-day cooking or you need some inspiration and a more structured approach to incorporating more variety into your family's meals, then this meal plan will help you to find your feet! And you don't need to worry about cooking from scratch for every single meal. This meal plan is reflective of the busy lives we lead, and makes space for rest and recuperation from cooking, which we all need. It's okay to take short cuts, and it's okay to take breaks from cooking. Burning ourselves out is never the answer, and there is a way to find balance and make space for respite while still prioritizing nutritious and tasty food.

What's more, you don't need to worry about trying to source a bunch of unusual ingredients that are hard to find or introducing too many new fruits and veggies at once. I have intentionally focused on meals and sides that use ingredients that are familiar and widely available and included a healthy dose of repetition because there is nothing wrong with repeating foods that are easily accessible to us and that our children enjoy. Variety is not just about the foods we serve, but how we serve them!

Lastly, following this meal plan may involve introducing a lot of new foods and recipes to your family, and toddlers in particular might find this challenging. I recommend starting slow and making adjustments where needed so that your toddler doesn't become overwhelmed. Feel free to include at least one preferred food in their meals so that your toddler can adjust comfortably and not feel pressured to eat foods they are not sure about or are still learning to like.

How the Meal Plan Works

When creating this meal plan, my main goal was to focus on striking a balance between making space in our day-to-day lives for creating nutritious home-cooked meals and being mindful of the busy lives we lead and the challenges we face looking after small children and keeping up with other responsibilities. We all have different circumstances, and it's impossible for me to cover all bases, but whether you are a working parent or a stay-at-home parent, this meal plan will give you some helpful tips and ideas on how you can incorporate the meals from this book into your everyday lives.

WEEKLY PLANS

The meal plans are each a week long, starting on a Monday. They are designed to follow each other, meaning that some of the meals you create will be utilized for leftovers later on, so you will cook less overall and save time.

You don't have to start each meal plan on a Monday, and you can absolutely switch around the days if that works better for you, but just be mindful that the meal plans are designed so that they can work within your work week and be reflective of the challenges you may face at different times during the week. Weekday meals are typically easier to prepare, quick and often make use of leftovers or foods that have been prepared previously, whereas the meals set out for the weekend are reflective of us having a little more time to prepare and cook meals and potentially having more help on hand. With that said, whichever way you decide to navigate the meal plan is fine, and what is going to be most helpful to you is whatever makes the most sense for your personal circumstances and family lifestyle.

FLEXIBLE DAYS

You will notice that on the weekend, there are certain meals marked as "flexible." This is to allow you to utilize leftovers should you have any, or make space for takeout, days out, visiting friends and family or just to have a breather from the meal plan and cook whatever you fancy or what your kids have requested. Feel free to add in more flexible meals on other days if that works for you but be sure to double check if the meals you are skipping will be needed for leftovers on another day and whether that will be more work for you.

BATCH COOKING

In order to make the meal plan work and to save you time and energy during the week, there is a small amount of batch cooking involved, which mostly involves easy-to-prep foods. Try and find an hour on the weekend to prepare these foods and store them for the week ahead so you can make the most out of this meal plan.

FRUIT & VEGGIE SUGGESTIONS

For many of the meals in the plan, I have included some specific fruit and vegetable suggestions that will complement the meal and help to keep things varied, but these are just suggestions. They can be switched out as needed, depending on your mood, the season and the affordability of the foods. Many fruits and vegetable are repeated, and this is okay. In real life, variety doesn't mean serving different things all the time, so serving the same things in different ways or in different combinations is perfectly fine and more realistic in practice. Not to mention, for many toddlers, repeated exposure is essential in helping them learn to like different fruits and vegetables.

LUNCHBOXES

Most of the lunches in the plan can be packed into a lunchbox, and for lunches that might be trickier to pack, I have provided an alternative. All the meals in the plan are nutritionally balanced, but feel free to add in whatever foods you feel are necessary for your child's lunchbox. When it comes to packing lunches for daycare or school, it's important to pack foods that your child will reliably eat. This means including familiar and preferred foods so that you know they will have nourishing options to keep them energized throughout the day. If you feel that the suggested lunch foods in this meal plan will not be eaten and your child will likely go hungry, do not hesitate to make swaps where needed. You can focus on introducing new foods at home and make adjustments for an uneaten lunch in their afternoon snack.

SNACKS

I haven't included snacks in this meal plan because I wanted to provide some space for flexibility and navigating the day-to-day changes in your toddler's appetite. Additionally, you can use snack time as an opportunity to include your toddlers favorite or preferred foods that may not be included in the meal plan. Be sure to check out Chapter 2 (page 26) for my guide to managing toddler snacks, and if you want specific snack ideas, you can find some Easy Balanced Snack examples on page 30.

MODIFICATIONS

Be sure to modify how you serve the foods in this meal plan according to your toddler's age and eating skills. I have provided some information on modifying common choking hazards in Chapter 1 in the Choking Hazard Guidelines section of this book (page 16), but please note that this list is not exhaustive. Please refer to current government guidelines for a comprehensive list.

Meal Plan Week 1

MEALS TO MAKE AHEAD

1. Toddler-Friendly Nut-Free Granola (page 38)
2. Lemon & Blueberry Yogurt Muffins (page 146)

	BREAKFAST	LUNCH & LUNCHBOX	DINNER
MONDAY	**Main:** Iron-Rich Banana & Cashew Oatmeal (page 54) **Sides:** Vitamin C-rich fruit, such as strawberries, oranges, kiwi	**Main:** Full-fat or nondairy cream cheese and hemp heart bagel **Sides:** Lemon & Blueberry Yogurt Muffin (page 146), cucumber and fruit of choice	**Main:** Speedy Cherry Tomato Spaghetti (page 85) **Optional Sides:** Store-bought garlic bread and grated parmesan
TUESDAY	**Main:** Fortified cereal (see notes) and full-fat or nondairy milk **Side:** Apple or banana	**Main:** Avocado Egg Salad (page 94) whole-grain sandwich **Sides:** Thinly sliced raw bell pepper and clementine	**Main:** Baked potatoes & toppings (see notes)
WEDNESDAY	**Main:** Easy Peachy Smoothie Bowl (page 46) **Sides:** Top with Toddler-Friendly Nut-Free Granola (page 38) and sliced banana	**Main:** 10-Minute Peanut Noodles (page 90) **Sides:** Julienned carrot, watermelon and a (optional) snack bar	**Main:** Hearty Mexican Chicken Quesadillas (page 71) **Side:** Buttered corn on the cob
THURSDAY	**Main:** Nut or seed butter toast & hemp hearts **Side:** Orange wedges	**Main:** Turkey & cheese tortilla roll-up **Sides:** Lemon & Blueberry Yogurt Muffin (page 146), cucumber and quartered red grapes	**Main:** Curried Lentil & Veggie Soup (page 82), see notes **Optional Side:** Buttered crusty bread or toast
FRIDAY	**Main:** Overnight oats (see notes) **Toppings:** Defrosted frozen fruit (see notes) and a (optional) drizzle of honey for kids 2+ years	**Main:** Leftover Curried Lentil & Veggie Soup **Side:** Ripe pear **Lunchbox Variation:** Mini charcuterie (see notes)	**Main:** Store-bought veggie or meat sausages **Sides:** Broccoli Mashed Potatoes (page 120) and cooked carrots
SATURDAY	**Main:** Broccoli & Cheese Sheet Pan Eggs (page 41, see notes) **Sides:** Buttered toasted English muffin and avocado	**FLEXIBLE**	**FLEXIBLE**
SUNDAY	**Main:** Whole-Wheat Protein Blender Waffles (page 37, see notes) **Sides:** Defrosted frozen blueberries	**FLEXIBLE**	**Main:** Crispy Salmon Bites (page 69, see notes) **Sides:** Cinnamon Roasted Sweet Potatoes (page 124) and cooked green peas

WEEK 1 NOTES

Fortified Cereal

Choose a fortified cereal with a few grams of fiber and protein and with little added sugar. This will help to keep toddlers going until snack time.

Baked Potatoes

How to cook: Scrub medium-sized baking potatoes and poke them multiple times with a fork. Rub the potatoes with oil and season with salt. Bake in the oven at 400°F (200°C, gas mark 6, fan 180°C) for 40 to 60 minutes, or until golden and tender. To serve, slit the top of the potatoes lengthwise and push each end of the potatoes to open them wide, or cut into roughly 1-inch (2.5-cm) pieces and top with butter (or nondairy alternative).

Here are some suggested toppings and sides:

Protein and/or Fat

- Grated cheese
- Baked beans
- Sour Cream
- Chopped crispy bacon
- Canned salmon or tuna and mayonnaise
- Coleslaw

Veggies

- Sweet corn
- Fresh sliced chives
- Shredded carrot
- Chopped tomatoes
- Chopped sautéed mushrooms
- Steamed veggies, such as broccoli or cauliflower
- Salad

Curried Lentil & Veggie Soup

Be sure to save the leftover soup, as you will need it for a quick lunch the next day. If you don't think you will have enough for leftovers, I recommend making a double batch.

Overnights Oats

How to make (serves 4): Combine 3 cups (720 ml) of milk and 3 cups (270 g) of rolled oats in a large container and mix until well combined. Cover and refrigerate overnight. When you are ready to serve, you may wish to add a little more milk to loosen up the oats to your desired consistency. Serve cold or warm.

Defrosted Frozen Fruit

Defrosting and warming frozen fruit in the microwave helps to release their natural juices and provide delicious natural sweetness for kids under 2 years old.

Mini Charcuterie

- Multigrain crackers or crackers of choice
- Cheddar cheese
- Smoked sausage
- Hummus
- Quartered cherry or grape tomatoes
- Sliced apple

Broccoli & Cheese Sheet Pan Eggs

Be sure to freeze the leftovers, as you will need them for a quick lunch next week. If you don't think you will have enough for leftovers, I recommend making a double batch.

Whole-Wheat Protein Blender Waffles

Be sure to freeze the leftovers, as you will need them for a quick breakfast next week. If you don't think you will have enough for leftovers, I recommend making a double batch.

Crispy Salmon Bites

Make a double batch of the Crispy Salmon Bites and freeze one batch before cooking—you will need this for Week 4 (page 160) of this meal plan. See the recipe for full freezing and storage instructions (page 69).

Meal Plan Week 2

MEALS TO MAKE AHEAD

1. Orange & Raspberry Muffins (page 131)
2. No-Bake Multigrain Cereal Bars (page 132)

	BREAKFAST	LUNCH & LUNCHBOX	DINNER
MONDAY	**Main:** Full-fat or nondairy plain yogurt **Sides:** Top with Toddler-Friendly Nut-Free Granola (page 38, see notes) and fresh or defrosted frozen mango	**Main:** Hummus and shredded carrot sandwich roll ups **Sides:** Orange & Raspberry Muffin (page 131), quartered cherry or grape tomatoes and an applesauce pot or pouch	**Main:** Stovetop Pumpkin Mac & Cheese (page 75) **Side:** Cooked broccoli
TUESDAY	**Main:** Boiled egg **Sides:** Buttered toast and banana	**Main:** Crispy Sweet Corn Fritters (page 98, see notes) **Sides:** Fried, scrambled or boiled egg, avocado (see notes) and pineapple (see notes)	**Main:** Lemony Chicken & Leek Sheet Pan (page 97) **Side:** Parmesan Crusted Roasties (page 115)
WEDNESDAY	**Main:** No-Bake Multigrain Cereal Bar (page 132) **Sides:** Full-fat or nondairy milk and sliced peaches (see notes)	**Main:** Cream cheese pasta (see notes) **Sides:** Edamame and fruit of choice **Lunchbox Variation:** Homemade Lunchables® (see notes)	**Main:** Sweet Potato Mini Pizzas (page 66) **Side:** Sautéed Green Beans (page 111)
THURSDAY	**Main:** Overnight oats (see notes) **Side:** Top with defrosted frozen fruit and a (optional) drizzle of honey for kids 2+ years	**Main:** Peanut butter & sliced strawberry sandwich **Sides:** Full-fat cottage cheese or nondairy plain yogurt, celery cut into matchsticks and cantaloupe melon	**Main:** Spinach & Cod Mild Coconut Curry (page 101) **Side:** Basmati rice
FRIDAY	**Main:** Freezer stash Whole-Wheat Protein Blender Waffles (page 37) made into waffle sandwiches using nut or seed butter of choice **Sides:** Full-fat or nondairy milk and raspberries	**Main:** Freezer stash Broccoli & Cheese Sheet Pan Eggs (page 41, see notes) **Sides:** Orange & Raspberry Muffin (page 131), cucumber, ranch dip and sliced plum	**Main:** Chunky Veggie Pasta Bake (page 102) **Side:** Store-bought garlic bread
SATURDAY	**Main:** Sweet Potato Breakfast Hash (page 49) **Side:** Scrambled, fried or boiled eggs	**FLEXIBLE**	**FLEXIBLE**
SUNDAY	**Main:** Fluffy Applesauce Pancakes (page 42, see notes) **Sides:** Full-fat Greek yogurt or plain yogurt of choice, fresh or defrosted frozen berries (see notes) and a (optional) drizzle of pure maple syrup for kids 2+ years	**FLEXIBLE**	**Main:** Lamb Kofta & Tzatziki Dip (page 76) **Sides:** Crispy Smoky Roasted Eggplant (page 123), flatbread, sliced tomatoes and shredded lettuce

WEEK 2 NOTES

Toddler-Friendly Nut-Free Granola

If you have run out of granola, you can pair the yogurt with fortified cereal instead.

Crispy Sweet Corn Fritters

If your toddler is having a lunchbox, I recommend making the fritters the night before.

Avocado

When packing avocado in a lunchbox, add a generous squeeze of lemon or lime juice to prevent browning and add flavor.

Pineapple

If fresh pineapple is hard to find or out of season, you can serve canned or jarred pineapple. Just be sure to choose pineapple that is preserved in juice, not syrup.

Sliced Peaches

If fresh peaches are hard to find or out of season, you can serve canned or jarred peaches. Just be sure to choose peaches that are preserved in juice, not syrup.

Cream Cheese Pasta

How to make (serves 4): Combine 14 ounces (400 g) of cooked pasta with ¼ cup (60 g) full-fat cream cheese or nondairy cream cheese of choice, a pinch of salt and black pepper and mix until well combined. Add more cream cheese if desired.

Homemade Lunchables

- Crackers
- Sliced cheese
- Low sodium salami
- Mild salsa (see tip)
- Shredded carrot
- Quartered grapes

Tip: When shopping for mild salsa, be sure to check out the chilled section at the supermarket as fresh varieties of salsa tend to have less added sugar and a ton more flavor.

Overnight Oats

How to make (serves 4): Combine 3 cups (720 ml) of milk and 3 cups (270 g) of rolled oats in a large container and mix until well combined. Cover and refrigerate overnight. When you are ready to serve, you may wish to add a little more milk to loosen up the oats to your desired consistency. Serve cold or warm.

Broccoli & Cheese Sheet Pan Eggs

If you don't have any leftovers on hand, you can serve a boiled egg instead.

Fluffy Applesauce Pancakes

Be sure to freeze the leftovers, as you will need them for a quick breakfast next week. If you don't think you will have enough for leftovers, I recommend making a double batch.

Defrosted Frozen Berries

Defrosting and warming frozen fruit in the microwave helps to release their natural juices and provide delicious natural sweetness for kids under 2 years old.

Meal Plan Week 3

MEALS TO MAKE AHEAD

1. Pumpkin Pie Mini Muffins (page 141)
2. Apple & Carrot Snack Bars (page 145)
3. Homemade Marinara Dipping Sauce (page 127)

	BREAKFAST	LUNCH & LUNCHBOX	DINNER
MONDAY	**Main:** Iron-Rich Banana & Cashew Oatmeal (page 54) **Side:** Vitamin C-rich fruit such as strawberries, oranges, kiwi	Mini charcuterie (see notes)	**Main:** 20-Minute Iron-Rich Tomato Soup (page 59, see notes) **Sides:** Cheesy Garlic Bread (page 108) and fruit or veggie of choice
TUESDAY	**Main:** Full-fat cream cheese (or nondairy cream cheese of choice) on whole-grain toast with hemp hearts **Side:** Blackberries	**Main:** 10-Minute Peanut Noodles (page 90) **Sides:** Cucumber, carrot matchsticks and applesauce pot or pouch	**Main:** Store-bought chicken tenders (see notes) **Sides:** Store-bought hash browns (see notes), Homemade Marinara Dipping Sauce (page 127) and Sautéed Green Beans (page 111)
WEDNESDAY	**Main:** Apple & Carrot Snack Bar (page 145) **Sides:** Full-fat Greek yogurt or plain yogurt of choice and pomegranate seeds.	**Main:** Leftover chicken tenders with mayonnaise and lettuce on a whole-grain wrap **Sides:** Avocado (see notes) and blueberries	**Main:** Shrimp Cakes (page 86) **Sides:** Crispy Zucchini Fries (page 107) and fruit of choice
THURSDAY	**Main:** Freezer stash Fluffy Applesauce Pancakes (page 42) made into pancake sandwiches using nut or seed butter **Sides:** Full-fat milk or nondairy milk and kiwi	**Main:** Cheesy Broccoli Balls (page 142, see notes) **Sides:** Homemade Marinara Dipping Sauce (page 127), pita bread and raspberries	**Main:** Meat or veggie sausages **Sides:** Parmesan Crusted Roasties (page 115) and buttered corn on the cob
FRIDAY	**Main:** Chia pudding (see notes) **Sides:** Fresh berries and a (optional) drizzle of honey for kids over 2 years old	**Main:** Cheese & tomato whole-grain sandwich **Sides:** Pumpkin Pie Mini Muffin (page 141) and fruit of choice	**Main:** Smoky Honey Chicken Drumsticks (page 60, see notes) **Sides:** Serve with store-bought potato wedges and veggie of choice
SATURDAY	**Main:** Savory Cheddar Waffles (page 53, see notes) **Sides:** Scrambled, fried or boiled egg and avocado	**FLEXIBLE**	**FLEXIBLE**
SUNDAY	**Main:** Breakfast Banana Cake Cups (page 50) **Sides:** Full-fat Greek yogurt or nondairy yogurt of choice and defrosted frozen cherries (see notes)	**FLEXIBLE**	**Main:** Oven-Baked Turkey & Spinach Meatballs (page 63) **Sides:** Easy Garlic Noodles (page 112), shredded parmesan cheese (optional) and cooked broccoli

WEEK 3 NOTES

Mini Charcuterie:
- Multigrain crackers or crackers of choice
- Cheddar cheese
- Smoked sausage
- Hummus
- Thinly sliced red bell pepper
- Clementine
- Pumpkin Pie Mini Muffin (page 141)

20-Minute Iron-Rich Tomato Soup
Make a double batch and freeze one batch after cooking—you will need this for a quick lunch on week 4 of this meal plan.

Chicken Tenders
Make more chicken tenders than you will need, as you will be using the leftovers for a quick lunch the next day.

Hash Browns
Many grocery stores carry a wide range of hash browns, including those with added veggies such as cauliflower, so don't be afraid to try new varieties if that is an option for you.

Avocado
When packing avocado in a lunchbox, add a generous squeeze of lemon or lime to prevent browning and add flavor.

Cheesy Broccoli Balls
- If your toddler is having a lunchbox, I recommend making the Cheesy Broccoli Balls the night before.
- Be sure to freeze the leftover Cheesy Broccoli Balls, as you will need them for a quick lunch next week. If you don't think you will have enough for leftovers, I recommend making a double batch.

Chia Pudding
How to make (serves 4): In a large container, combine 1 cup (240 ml) of full-fat milk or milk of choice, 1 cup (280 g) of full-fat plain Greek yogurt and ¼ cup (40 g) of chia seeds and mix until well combined. Cover and refrigerate for 30 minutes and then mix again. Cover and return to the refrigerator overnight.

Smoky Honey Chicken Drumsticks
Honey must not be served to babies under 1 due to the risk of infant botulism.

Savory Cheddar Waffles
Be sure to freeze the leftover waffles, as you will need them for a quick lunch next week. If you don't think you will have enough for leftovers, I recommend making a double batch.

Defrosted Frozen Cherries
Defrosting and warming frozen cherries in the microwave helps to release their natural juices and provide delicious natural sweetness to complement the yogurt.

Meal Plan Week 4

MEALS TO MAKE AHEAD

1. Lemon & Blueberry Yogurt Muffins (page 146)
2. Lemon Garlic Dip (page 116)

	BREAKFAST	LUNCH & LUNCHBOX	DINNER
MONDAY	**Main:** Boiled egg **Sides:** Avocado toast with hulled hemp hearts, fruit of choice	**Main:** Falafel Patties (page 89, see notes) **Sides:** Lemon Garlic Dip (page 116), cucumber, sliced plum and a store-bought snack bar	**Main:** Freezer stash Crispy Salmon Bites (page 69) **Sides:** Broccoli Mashed Potatoes (page 120) and cooked carrots
TUESDAY	**Main:** Easy Peachy Smoothie Bowl (page 46) **Side:** Lemon & Blueberry Yogurt Muffin (page 146)	**Main:** Freezer stash Cheesy Broccoli Balls (page 142) **Sides:** Mild salsa (see notes), crackers, apple chips and quartered green grapes	**Main:** Meat or veggie burger with buns and preferred fillings (see notes) **Side:** Crispy Zucchini Fries (page 107)
WEDNESDAY	**Main:** Fortified cereal (see notes) & full fat milk or nondairy milk **Side:** Sliced banana	**Main:** Leftover burger **Sides:** Easy Garlic Noodles (page 112), cooked green peas and fruit of choice	Mexican baked sweet potatoes & toppings (see notes)
THURSDAY	**Main:** Overnight oats (see notes) **Sides:** Top with defrosted frozen berries (see notes) and a (optional) drizzle of honey for kids over 2 years old	**Main:** Freezer stash 20-Minute Iron-Rich Tomato Soup (page 59) **Sides:** Cheesy Garlic Bread (page 108) and fruit or veggie of choice **Lunchbox Variation:** Nut or seed butter & sliced strawberry whole-grain sandwich, Lemon & Blueberry Yogurt Muffin (page 146), carrot matchsticks and cucumber	**Main:** Quick-Cook Sausage & Pepper Stew (page 93, see notes) **Side:** Eggy Bread Rolls (page 119)
FRIDAY	**Main:** Freezer stash Savory Cheddar Waffles (page 53) **Sides:** Boiled egg and grapefruit	**Main:** Leftover Quick-Cook Sausage & Pepper Stew (page 93) on a sub or roll **Sides:** Full-fat Greek yogurt or nondairy yogurt of choice and ripe pear	**Main:** Speedy Cherry Tomato Spaghetti (page 85) **Sides:** Cooked snap peas and shredded parmesan
SATURDAY	**Main:** Broccoli & Cheese Sheet Pan Eggs (page 41) **Sides:** Toasted English whole-grain muffin and kiwi	**FLEXIBLE**	**FLEXIBLE**
SUNDAY	**Main:** Blueberry & Banana French Toast Bake (page 45, see notes) **Side:** Greek or nondairy yogurt or whipped cream	**FLEXIBLE**	**Main:** Lazy Lasagna Soup (page 79) **Side:** Fruit or veggie of choice

WEEK 4 NOTES

Falafel Patties

If your toddler is having a lunchbox, I recommend making the Falafel Patties the night before.

Salsa

When shopping for mild salsa, be sure to check out the chilled section at the supermarket as fresh varieties of salsa tend to have less added sugar and a ton more flavor.

Burgers

- Serve the burgers deconstructed for younger toddlers who may find assembled burgers challenging to eat.
- Make more burger patties than you will need, as you will be using them for a quick lunch the next day.

Fortified Cereal

When choosing a fortified cereal, look for options with a few grams of fiber and protein and with little added sugar. This will help to keep toddlers going until snack time.

Mexican Baked Sweet Potatoes:

How to cook: Scrub large sweet potatoes and poke them multiple times with a fork. Rub the potatoes with oil and season with salt. Bake in the oven at 400°F (200°C, gas mark 6, fan 180°C) for 35 to 45 minutes, or until golden and a knife can be inserted into the center of the potatoes without resistance. To serve, slit the top of the potatoes lengthwise and push each end of the potatoes to open them wide, or cut into roughly 1-inch pieces and top with butter or nondairy alternative.

Here are some suggested toppings for the sweet potatoes:

Protein and/or Fat

- Shredded cheese
- Kidney or black beans
- Refried beans
- Sour Cream
- Chopped crispy bacon
- Butter

Veggies

- Mild salsa
- Mild guacamole or mashed avocado with lime
- Sweet corn
- Fresh sliced chives
- Shredded carrot
- Chopped sautéed mushrooms
- Red bell pepper—cooked or raw
- Sliced scallions
- Fresh chopped cilantro

Overnight Oats:

How to make (serves 4): Combine 3 cups (720 ml) of milk and 3 cups (270 g) of rolled oats in a large container and mix until well combined. Cover and refrigerate overnight. When you are ready to serve, you may wish to add a little more milk to loosen up the oats to your desired consistency. Serve cold or warm.

Defrosted Frozen Berries

Defrosting and warming frozen fruit in the microwave helps to release their natural juices and provide delicious natural sweetness for kids under 2 years old.

Quick-Cook Sausage & Pepper Stew

Be sure to save the leftover stew, as you will need it for a quick lunch the next day. If you don't think you will have enough for leftovers, I recommend making a double batch.

Blueberry & Banana French Toast Bake

For best results and quicker breakfast prep, prepare (but don't cook) the Blueberry & Banana French Toast Bake the night before.

American/British Ingredient Translations

AMERICAN	BRITISH
Heavy cream	Double cream
Scallion/green onion	Spring onions
All-purpose flour	Plain flour
Whole-wheat flour	Wholemeal flour
Zucchini	Courgette
Ground meat	Minced meat
Grape tomatoes	Plum tomatoes
Eggplant	Aubergine
Almond meal	Ground almonds

Acknowledgments

A massive thank you to my community at Zayne's Plate. Your unwavering support of my work has been a huge motivator for me to continue doing what I do so passionately. Without you, none of this would have ever been possible, and I am forever grateful for your love and support over the past 6 years!

A special thank you to my five wonderful children who have made me the cook I am today—everything I make is always with you in mind and you have been the best (and always brutally honest) taste testers.

To Dean, thank you for always supporting me and reminding me that I can achieve anything I want, and of course for giving up so much of your time so that I could work on this amazing book.

To my editor Sarah Monroe at Page Street Publishing, thank you for giving me another opportunity to create a book that has allowed me to showcase my recipes to the fullest. As always, it's been a pleasure working with you and your input is invaluable.

About the Author

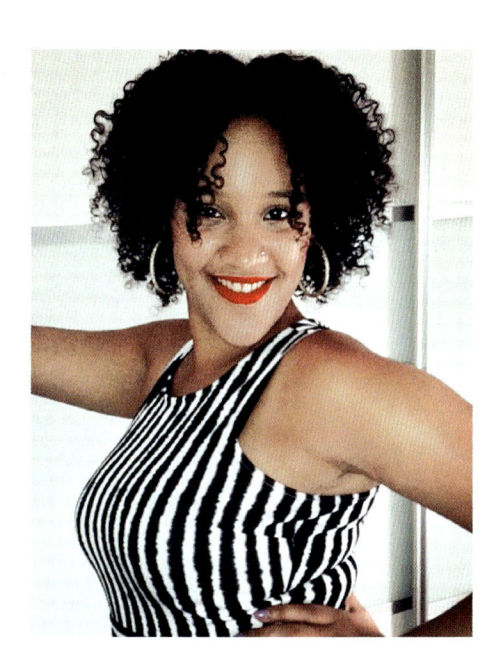

Simone Ward is a mom of five, a food writer and the creator of Zayne's Plate, a popular baby, toddler and kid feeding blog that helps parents to feed their families a wide variety of easy, healthy and tasty meals, as well as provides tips for supporting young children in having a healthy relationship with food. Having worked extensively in recipe development for a number of years, Simone specializes in creating nutritious family-friendly food for clients both domestically and internationally.

Simone's work has been featured on various websites, including The Everymom® article "8 Instagram Accounts That Make Feeding Toddlers Way Easier" that highlights Simone's simple yet nutritious meal ideas that appeal to toddlers and expand their culinary horizons.

Index

A

Age suitability, 21

Almond meal
- Crispy Zucchini Fries, 107
- Iron-Rich Almond & Coconut Cookies, 138

American/British ingredient translations, 162

Appetite, of toddlers, 11

Apples, 17
- Apple & Carrot Snack Bars, 145

Applesauce
- Fluffy Applesauce Pancakes, 42
- No-Bake Multigrain Cereal Bars, 132–134
- Toddler-Friendly Nut-Free Granola, 38

Avocado, in Avocado Egg salad, 94

B

Baby carrots, 17

Bacon, in Sweet Potato Breakfast Hash, 49

Baked potatoes, 155

Banana(s)
- Apple & Carrot Snack Bars, 145
- Blueberry & Banana French Toast Bake, 45
- Breakfast Banana Cake Cups, 50
- Easy Peachy Smoothie Bowl, 46
- Iron-Rich Banana & Cashew Oatmeal, 54
- Whole-Wheat Protein Blender Waffles, 37

Basil, fresh
- Speedy Cherry Tomato Spaghetti, 85
- 20-Minute Iron-Rich Tomato Soup, 59

Batch cooking, 153

Beans, 32, 161
- 20-Minute Iron-Rich Tomato Soup, 59

Bedtime snacks, 29

Beef, in Lazy Lasagna Soup, 79–81

Bell pepper, 31
- Chunky Veggie Pasta Bake, 102
- Hearty Mexican Chicken Quesadillas, 71–72
- Lazy Lasagna Soup, 79–81
- Quick-Cook Sausage & Pepper Stew, 93
- Sweet Potato Breakfast Hash, 49

Berries, 17. *See also* Blueberries
- Bite-Size Fruity Cheesecake Strudels, 135–137
- Breakfast Banana Cake Cups, 50
- defrosting frozen, 155, 157, 159, 161
- Orange & Raspberry Muffins, 131

Blackberries, 17

Blueberries, 17
- Blueberry & Banana French Toast Bake, 45
- Lemon & Blueberry Yogurt Muffins, 146

Bread(s), 31
- Blueberry & Banana French Toast Bake, 45
- Cheesy Garlic Bread, 108

Breadcrumbs. *See* Panko breadcrumbs

Bread Rolls, Eggy, 119

Breakfast, in meal plans, 154, 156, 158, 160

Breastfeeding, 21

Bribery, picky eating and, 13

Brioche bread, in Blueberry & Banana French Toast Bake, 45

British/American ingredient translations, 162

Broccoli, 31
- Broccoli & Cheese Sheet Pan Eggs, 41
- Broccoli Mashed Potatoes, 120
- Cheesy Broccoli Balls, 142

Burgers, 161

Butternut squash, in Curried Lentil & Veggie Soup, 82

C

Carrots, 17
- Apple & Carrot Snack Bars, 145
- Chunky Veggie Pasta Bake, 102
- Curried Lentil & Veggie Soup, 82

Cashew butter, in Iron-Rich Banana & Cashew Oatmeal, 54

Celery, 17

Cereal
- fortified, 155, 161
- No-Bake Multigrain Cereal Bars, 132–134

Charcuterie, mini, 155, 159

Cheddar cheese
- Broccoli & Cheese Sheet Pan Eggs, 41
- Cheesy Broccoli Balls, 142
- Savory Cheddar Waffles, 53
- Stovetop Pumpkin Mac & Cheese, 75

Cheese, 17. *See also* specific cheeses
- Chunky Veggie Pasta Bake, 102

Cherries, 17, 159

Cherry tomatoes
- Chunky Veggie Pasta Bake, 102
- Speedy Cherry Tomato Spaghetti, 85

Chia seeds
- Bite-Size Fruity Cheesecake Strudels, 135–137
- Chia Pudding, 159

Chicken
- Hearty Mexican Chicken Quesadillas, 71–72
- Lemony Chicken & Leek Sheet Pan, 97
- Smoky Honey Chicken Drumsticks, 60–62

Chickpea pasta, in Stovetop Pumpkin Mac & Cheese, 75

Chickpeas
- Cheesy Broccoli Balls, 142
- Falafel Patties, 89

Chives
- Eggy Bread Rolls, 119
- Sweet Potato Breakfast Hash, 49

Chocolate chips, in Breakfast Banana Cake Cups, 50

Chocolate Oat Bites, 149

Choking hazards, 16–18

Cocoa powder, in Chocolate Oat Bites, 149

Coconut
- Iron-Rich Almond & Coconut Cookies, 138
- Toddler-Friendly Nut-Free Granola, 38

Coconut milk, in Spinach & Cod Mild Coconut Curry, 101

Cod, in Spinach & Cod Mild Coconut Curry, 101

Cookies, Iron-Rich Almond & Coconut, 138

Corn, 17
- Crispy Sweet Corn Fritters, 98

Cow milk, 21

Cream cheese
- Bite-Size Fruity Cheesecake Strudels, 135–137
- Cream Cheese Pasta, 157
- Stovetop Pumpkin Mac & Cheese, 75

Cucumber, in Lamb Kofta & Tzatziki Dip, 76–78

Curried Lentil & Veggie Soup, 82

Cutlery, encouraging your toddler to use, 22

D

Desserts, 19–21

Dips
- Homemade Marinara Dipping Sauce, 127
- Lemon Garlic Dip, 116

Divided plates, 22

Division of Responsibility (DoR), 12–13, 121

E

Egg(s)
- Avocado Egg Salad, 94
- Blueberry & Banana French Toast Bake, 45
- Breakfast Banana Cake Cups, 50
- Broccoli & Cheese Sheet Pan Eggs, 41
- Cheesy Broccoli Balls, 142
- Crispy Salmon Bites, 69–70
- Crispy Sweet Corn Fritters, 98
- Crispy Zucchini Fries, 107
- Eggy Bread Rolls, 119
- Lemon & Blueberry Yogurt Muffins, 146
- Orange & Raspberry Muffins, 131
- Oven-Baked Turkey & Spinach Meatballs, 63–65
- Pumpkin Pie Mini Muffins, 141
- Savory Cheddar Waffles, 53
- Shrimp Cakes, 86
- snacking on, 32
- Whole-Wheat Protein Blender Waffles, 37

Eggplant
- Chunky Veggie Pasta Bake, 102
- Crispy Smoky Roasted Eggplant, 123

F

Falafel Patties, 89

Fish and seafood
- Crispy Salmon Bites, 69–70
- Shrimp Cakes, 86
- Spinach & Cod Mild Coconut Curry, 101

Flaxseed
- No-Bake Multigrain Cereal Bars, 132–134
- Whole-Wheat Protein Blender Waffles, 37

Food(s)
- snacking, 30, 31–32
- that are choking hazards, 17–18
- throwing, 24–25

Food games, 16

French Toast Bake, Blueberry & Banana, 45

Fritters, Crispy Sweet Corn, 98

Fruit(s). *See also* specific fruits
- defrosting frozen, 155, 157, 159, 161
- prepping, 29
- for snacking, 28, 31–32

G

Gagging, 16

Granola, Toddler-Friendly Nut-Free, 38

Grapes, 17

Grape tomatoes, 17
- Chunky Veggie Pasta Bake, 102
- Speedy Cherry Tomato Spaghetti, 85

Green Beans, Sautéed, 111

Green onions. *See* Scallions (green onions)

Ground beef, in Lazy Lasagna Soup, 79–81

Ground lamb, in Lamb Kofta & Tzatziki Dip, 76–78

Ground pork, in Lazy Lasagna Soup, 79–81

Ground turkey, in Oven-Baked Turkey & Spinach Meatballs, 63–65

H

Hands, toddlers eating with their, 22

Hard candy, 17

Hemp hearts
- Apple & Carrot Snack Bars, 145
- Chocolate Oat Bites, 149
- Iron-Rich Banana & Cashew Oatmeal, 54
- Toddler-Friendly Nut-Free Granola, 38

High chairs, 23–24

Hot dogs, 17

K

Kale, in Curried Lentil & Veggie Soup, 82

L

Lamb Kofta & Tzatziki Dip, 76–78

Leeks, in Lemony Chicken & Leek Sheet Pan, 97

Lemon
- Lemon & Blueberry Yogurt Muffins, 146
- Lemon Garlic Dip, 118
- Lemony Chicken & Leek Sheet Pan, 97

Lemon Garlic Dip
- recipe, 116
- Shrimp Cakes, 86

Lentil pasta, in Stovetop Pumpkin Mac & Cheese, 75

Lentils, in Curried Lentil & Veggie Soup, 82

Lunchboxes, 153

Lunch meal plans, 154, 156, 158, 160

M

Mac & Cheese, Stovetop Pumpkin, 75

Maple syrup
- Bite-Size Fruity Cheesecake Strudels, 135–137
- Homemade Marinara Dipping Sauce, 127
- Iron-Rich Almond & Coconut Cookies, 138
- Lemon & Blueberry Yogurt Muffins, 146
- Pumpkin Pie Mini Muffins, 141

Marinara Dipping Sauce, 127

Marshmallows, 17

Meal plans, 152–161

Mealtime schedules, 13, 30

Meatballs, Oven-Baked Turkey & Spinach, 63–65

Medjool dates, in Chocolate Oat Bites, 149

Messy eating, 15

Milk
- picky eating and, 13
- recommended amounts, 21
- what to do when your child will not drink, 21–22

Mozzarella cheese
- Cheesy Garlic Bread, 108
- Hearty Mexican Chicken Quesadillas, 71–72
- Sweet Potato Mini Pizzas, 66

Muffins
- Lemon & Blueberry Yogurt Muffins, 146
- Orange & Raspberry Muffins, 131
- Pumpkin Pie Mini Muffins, 141

Multigrain Cereal Bars, No-Bake, 132–134

N

Noodles
- Easy Garlic Noodles, 112
- 10-Minute Peanut Noodles, 90

Nut butter, 17, 31. *See also* Peanut butter
- Chocolate Oat Bites, 149
- Iron-Rich Banana & Cashew Oatmeal, 54
- No-Bake Multigrain Cereal Bars, 132–134

Nutritional yeast
- Crispy Salmon Bites, 69–70
- Crispy Zucchini Fries, 107
- Oven-Baked Turkey & Spinach Meatballs, 63–65
- Speedy Cherry Tomato Spaghetti, 85

Nuts, 17, 31. *See also* Nut butter; Peanut butter

O

Oatmeal, Iron-Rich Banana & Cashew, 54

Oats. *See* Rolled oats

Olives, 17

Orange juice/orange zest
- Easy Peachy Smoothie Bowl, 46
- Orange & Raspberry Muffins, 131

Overnight Oats, 155, 157, 161

P

Pancakes, Fluffy Applesauce, 42

Pancetta, in Sweet Potato Breakfast Hash, 49

Panko breadcrumbs
- Cheesy Broccoli Balls, 142
- Crispy Salmon Bites, 69–70
- Crispy Zucchini Fries, 107
- Lamb Kofta & Tzatziki Dip, 76–78
- Oven-Baked Turkey & Spinach Meatballs, 63–65
- Shrimp Cakes, 86

Parmesan cheese
- Crispy Salmon Bites, 69–70
- Crispy Zucchini Fries, 107
- Lazy Lasagna Soup, 79–81
- Oven-Baked Turkey & Spinach Meatballs, 63–65
- Parmesan Crusted Roasties, 115
- Speedy Cherry Tomato Spaghetti, 85

Parsley, fresh
- Cheesy Garlic Bread, 108
- Easy Garlic Noodles, 112
- Falafel Patties, 89
- Lazy Lasagna Soup, 79–81

Passata
- Chunky Veggie Pasta Bake, 102
- Hearty Mexican Chicken Quesadillas, 71–72
- Lazy Lasagna Soup, 79–81
- Oven-Baked Turkey & Spinach Meatballs, 63–65
- Sweet Potato Mini Pizzas, 66

Pasta dishes
- Chunky Veggie Pasta Bake, 102
- Cream Cheese Pasta, 157
- Easy Garlic Noodles, 112
- Lazy Lasagna Soup, 79–81
- Speedy Cherry Tomato Spaghetti, 85
- Stovetop Pumpkin Mac & Cheese, 75
- 10-Minute Peanut Noodles, 90

Peaches
- Easy Peachy Smoothie Bowl, 46
- using canned or jarred, 157

Peanut butter
- No-Bake Multigrain Cereal Bars, 132–134
- 10-Minute Peanut Noodles, 90

Pears, 17
Peas, 18
    Lemony Chicken & Leek Sheet Pan, 97
Picky eating, 11–15
Pineapple, 157
Pizzas, Sweet Potato Mini, 66
Plant-based milk, 21
Plates, divided vs. open, 23
Popcorn, 17
Portion sizes, 13, 21
Potatoes
    baked, 155
    Broccoli Mashed Potatoes, 120
    Parmesan Crusted Roasties, 115
Pressure strategies, picky eating and, 13–14
Protein, offering snacks high in, 28, 31–32
Puff pastry, in Bite-Size Fruity Cheesecake Strudels, 135–137
Pumpkin puree
    Pumpkin Pie Mini Muffins, 141
    Stovetop Pumpkin Mac & Cheese, 75

Q
Quesadillas, Hearty Mexican Chicken, 71–72

R
Raisins
    Breakfast Banana Cake Cups, 50
    Toddler-Friendly Nut-Free Granola, 38
Raspberries, 17
    Bite-Size Fruity Cheesecake Strudels, 135–137
    Orange & Raspberry Muffins, 131
Reward, sweets and desserts as a, 19
Ricotta cheese, in Lazy Lasagna Soup, 79–81
Rolled oats
    Apple & Carrot Snack Bars, 145
    Breakfast Banana Cake Cups, 50
    Chocolate Oat Bites, 149
    Iron-Rich Banana & Cashew Oatmeal, 54
    Overnight Oats, 155, 157, 161
    Toddler-Friendly Nut-Free Granola, 38
    Whole-Wheat Protein Blender Waffles, 37

S
Safe foods, 14
Salmon, in Crispy Salmon Bites, 69–70
Satter, Ellen, 12
Sausages, 17
    Quick-Cook Sausage & Pepper Stew, 93
Scallions (green onions)
    Cheesy Broccoli Balls, 142
    Crispy Sweet Corn Fritters, 98
    Falafel Patties, 89
    Shrimp Cakes, 86
    Spinach & Cod Mild Coconut Curry, 101
Scheduling snacks, 28, 29
Seed butter, 17, 31
    Chocolate Oat Bites, 149
    No-Bake Multigrain Cereal Bars, 132–134
Seeds, 31
Shrimp, in Shrimp Cakes, 86
Sieved tomatoes. *See* Passata
Smoothie Bowl, Easy Peachy, 46
Snack(s) and snack time, 153
    bedtime, 29
    foods that create balanced, 31–32
    formula for building, 28
    importance of, 27
    mini meals as, 27–28
    picky eating and, 13
    quick & easy "throw together," 30
    recipes, 30
    scheduling, 28, 29
    tips for stress-free, 29–30
    what is considered a nutritious, 27

Soups and stews
    Curried Lentil & Veggie Soup, 82
    Lazy Lasagna Soup, 79–81
    Quick-Cook Sausage & Pepper Stew, 93
    20-Minute Iron-Rich Tomato Soup, 59
Spinach
    Oven-Baked Turkey & Spinach Meatballs, 63–65
    Spinach & Cod Mild Coconut Curry, 101
Strawberries, in Bite-Size Fruity Cheesecake Strudels, 135–137
String cheese, 17
Sugar intake, introducing and managing, 18–21
Sunflower seed butter, in No-Bake Multigrain Cereal Bars, 132–134
Sunflower seeds, in Toddler-Friendly Nut-Free Granola, 38
Sweet potatoes
    Cinnamon Roasted Sweet Potatoes, 124
    Mexican Baked Sweet Potatoes, 161
    Sweet Potato Breakfast Hash, 49
    Sweet Potato Mini Pizzas, 66

T
Teething, picky eating and, 14
Throwing food, 24–25
Tiredness, picky eating and, 14
Toddler development, picky eating and, 12
Tomatoes, canned
    Curried Lentil & Veggie Soup, 82
    Homemade Marinara Dipping Sauce, 127
    Lazy Lasagna Soup, 79–81
    Oven-Baked Turkey & Spinach Meatballs, 63–65
    Quick-Cook Sausage & Pepper Stew, 93
    Sweet Potato Mini Pizzas, 66
    20-Minute Iron-Rich Tomato Soup, 59

Tomatoes, fresh. *See* Cherry tomatoes; Grape tomatoes

Tomatoes, strained
- Hearty Mexican Chicken Quesadillas, 71–72
- Sweet Potato Mini Pizzas, 66

Tomato paste
- Chunky Veggie Pasta Bake, 102
- Lazy Lasagna Soup, 79–81
- Oven-Baked Turkey & Spinach Meatballs, 63–65
- Quick-Cook Sausage & Pepper Stew, 93
- Speedy Cherry Tomato Spaghetti, 85
- Spinach & Cod Mild Coconut Curry, 101
- Sweet Potato Mini Pizzas, 66
- 20-Minute Iron-Rich Tomato Soup, 59

Tortillas, in Hearty Mexican Chicken Quesadillas, 71–72

V

Variety of foods, exposing toddler to a, 14, 22, 28, 152

Vegetables. *See also* specific vegetables
- prepping, 29
- repeated exposure to, 153
- for snacking, 28, 31–32

W

Waffles
- Savory Cheddar Waffles, 53
- Whole-Wheat Protein Blender Waffles, 37

Weekends, 152, 153

Weekly meal plans, 152–161

Y

Yogurt, 31
- Avocado Egg salad, 94
- Easy Peachy Smoothie Bowl, 46
- Lamb Kofta & Tzatziki Dip, 76–78
- Lemon & Blueberry Yogurt Muffins, 146
- Lemon Garlic Dip, 116
- Savory Cheddar Waffles, 53
- Whole-Wheat Protein Blender Waffles, 37

Z

Zucchini
- Chunky Veggie Pasta Bake, 102
- Crispy Zucchini Fries, 107